STUDENT WORKBOOK

DIMENSIONS OF
HUMAN SEXUALITY

Byer / Shainberg • *Third Edition*

DEBORAH A. MILLER
College of Charleston

Wm. C. Brown Publishers

This book is dedicated to my loving family. Thank you, Mom and Dad, Dave and Cindy, and Buffie and Schnaupps for all of your patience, understanding, and encouragement in this endeavor.

Cover illustration by Robert Phillips

ISBN 0–697–10070–7

Printed in the United States of America by Wm. C. Brown Publishers
2460 Kerper Boulevard, Dubuque, IA 52001

10 9 8 7 6 5 4

Contents

Preface

The *Dimensions of Human Sexuality* Student Workbook has been written to challenge your sexual being. Its introspective approach is designed for you to assess your sexual behaviors, attitudes, and feelings. But keep in mind that your behaviors, attitudes, and feelings may conflict at various times.

Each chapter is divided into four sections. The first section, comprised of various activities, should be completed *before* you read the related chapter in the textbook. These thought-provoking activities are designed to test your current level of knowledge and give you some insight into your personal values. *After* reading the chapter, you should attempt the second section, entitled "Reviewing Important Concepts." If you can answer these questions and understand the concepts, then you should go on to the third section entitled "Self-Discovery." This section may ask you to look to the past or the present or project yourself into the future to answer a question, situation, or social issue. There are no right or wrong answers in the Self-Discovery section, but you may want to compare your answers with those of your close friends. The final section, entitled "Self-Quizzes," reviews all of the material presented in the chapter. If you can answer these questions correctly, then you should do very well on the exam covering this material.

If you attempt to use this workbook with openness and honesty, the rewards can be immeasurable. It can foster a better understanding of your own sexuality and provide a springboard for you to understand the sexuality of your partner and others. Enjoy discovering your sexual self.

Acknowledgments

Some of the activities and questions found in this book are based on the innermost feelings shared with me by my friends. Their thoughts, fantasies, and fears challenged me to write this book in such a manner that we could search for the answers together.

I would like to thank from the bottom of my heart Dana and Joe Espinosa, Marsha Hass, Twitty Meyer, and Tommy Penninger for their insights and contributions.

1 Introduction to Human Sexuality

The narrowest description of your personhood occurred at your birth, when the doctor exclaimed, "It's a boy!" or "It's a girl!" Although these three words gave a clue as to your sex, it did not begin to tell who you would become or why. The term *sexuality* is a much broader term than the word *sex*. It refers not only to reproduction and the pursuit of sexual pleasure but also to the need for love and personal fulfillment. Sexuality incorporates the many psychological and cultural factors found in human sexual behavior.

What's Your Opinion?

Complete the following questionnaire by indicating the degree to which you agree or disagree with each of the statements, using the scale below. There are no correct or incorrect responses to these statements. After you have completed the questionnaire, try to determine why you answered the statements the way you did.

Strongly Agree	Agree	Disagree	Strongly Disagree
1	2	3	4

1. I have many close friends of the opposite sex.   1 2 3 4

2. When I hear the word *sex*, the first thing I think of is intercourse.   1 2 3 4

3. It doesn't take much to get me excited sexually.   1 2 3 4

4. If a woman asks a man out on a date, then she should pay all the expenses.   1 2 3 4

5. I am confident that a new sex partner would volunteer to tell me if he or she had been possibly exposed to a sexually transmitted disease.   1 2 3 4

6. Premarital sex is acceptable to me as long as there is a commitment between the individuals.   1 2 3 4

7. Before a couple can receive a marriage license, they should be required to have a blood test for AIDS.   1 2 3 4

8. Birth control is ultimately the woman's responsibility, as she is the one who gets pregnant.   1 2 3 4

9. Men should be free to express their emotions as openly as women.   1 2 3 4

10. It is important for me to reach orgasm each time my partner and I have intimate sexual relations.   1 2 3 4

11. Sexual fantasies should be shared with one's partner.   1 2 3 4

12. Lesbian behavior is more acceptable to me than similar behavior between gay men.   1 2 3 4

13. The incidence of oral sex is not rising; people are just more willing to talk about it.   1 2 3 4

14. If a woman says no to sex, she really means maybe. Therefore, the man should be more aggressive.   1 2 3 4

15. The decision to have an abortion should be made by the woman and her doctor, without the legal system being involved.   1 2 3 4

16. Sex education leads to experimentation and increased sexual activity.   1 2 3 4

17. Morality cannot be legislated and enforced.   1 2 3 4

18. The availability and accessibility of pornography has led to an increase in violent crimes.   1 2 3 4

19. Love without sex is unfulfilling.   1 2 3 4

20. It would be difficult for me to seek therapy for a sexual dysfunction.   1 2 3 4

21. Honest and open communication is the most important ingredient in a relationship.   1 2 3 4

22. Masturbation is a normal part of the sexual maturation process.   1 2 3 4

23. The thought of anal intercourse is exciting to me.   1 2 3 4

24. A married couple should have separate bank accounts in order to keep some autonomy in their lives.   1 2 3 4

25. It is important to me that when my partner and I have intimate sexual relations they be gentle and unhurried.   1 2 3 4

26. I would fake orgasm with my partner rather than hurt his or her feelings.   1 2 3 4

27. The majority of women suffer from premenstrual syndrome (PMS).   1 2 3 4

28. Men experience a change of life comparable to menopause in women.   1 2 3 4

29. I feel uncomfortable when I make noise during lovemaking.   1 2 3 4

30. I would like to experience both homosexual and heterosexual relationships.   1 2 3 4

31. It is difficult for me to tell my partner what I like or don't like about our lovemaking.   1 2 3 4

32. I feel sexually less experienced than most of my friends.   1 2 3 4

33. I would break up with my partner if I discovered that he or she had had sexual relations with someone else.   1 2 3 4

34. I feel uncomfortable initiating the sexual act.   1 2 3 4

35. Without saying a word, I generally know how my partner is feeling by his or her body language.   1 2 3 4

36. Convicted rapists should receive a mandatory twenty-year jail sentence without parole.   1 2 3 4

37. I would withhold sex from my partner as punishment for something he or she had done.   1 2 3 4

38. A couple should put up with an unhappy marriage for the sake of the children.   1 2 3 4

39. Touching another person is a major form of communication for me.   1 2 3 4

40. It excites me when I see an older couple in the park holding hands and kissing.   1 2 3 4

41. When my partner and I have a disagreement, we argue and yell, but the problem is resolved before one of us leaves.   1 2 3 4

42. In my opinion, there are some sexual acts that should remain illegal.   1 2 3 4

43. If my partner wanted to try a new position or technique during our lovemaking, I would find it exciting.   1 2 3 4

44. Prostitution should be decriminalized and legalized.   1 2 3 4

45. Notifying a minor's parents that he or she has been treated in a public health clinic would stop the minor from seeking treatment for a sexually transmitted disease.   1 2 3 4

46. Nurse-midwives are qualified practitioners to deliver a baby.   1 2 3 4

47. Men should be expected to change their last name when they get married.   1 2 3 4

48. Androgynous individuals express whatever behavior is appropriate in a given situation and disregard traditional sex roles.   1 2 3 4

49. Observing a couple in a public place touching each other is sexually stimulating to me.   1 2 3 4

50. Any sexual activity between consenting adults should be acceptable and legal.   1 2 3 4

51. Extramarital sexual intercourse is unacceptable under any circumstance.   1 2 3 4

52. Penis or breast size is irrelevant to sexual pleasure.   1 2 3 4

53. Living together is a viable alternative to marriage for me.   1 2 3 4

54. It is important for me to have some time alone each day.   1 2 3 4

55. I feel comfortable about the ways I choose to express myself sexually.   1 2 3 4

56. Males have fewer erogenous zones than females.   1 2 3 4

57. Aphrodisiacs are effective in increasing sexual pleasure.   1 2 3 4

58. A double standard still exists for male and female sexual behavior.   1 2 3 4

59. Sometimes I am embarrassed by my behavior on a date.   1 2 3 4

60. I feel that I am sexually very attractive.   1 2 3 4

61. I have fantasized about being involved in a sex orgy.   1 2 3 4

62. My religious upbringing has had a significant impact on my sexual values.   1 2 3 4

63. Although I love my partner very much, he or she does not satisfy all of my physical and emotional needs.   1 2 3 4

64. It was a shock the first time I realized that my parents were sexually active.   1 2 3 4

65. I could be romantically involved with a partner of a different racial background.   1 2 3 4

66. I would feel uncomfortable being seen in a gay bar.   1 2 3 4

67. It would be very difficult for me to adapt to my partner's becoming physically disabled.   1 2 3 4

68. Mate swapping is disgusting to me.   1 2 3 4

69. I would be jealous if I saw my partner having lunch with a member of the opposite sex.   1 2 3 4

70. I feel rejected if I do not have a date on Friday or Saturday night.   1 2 3 4

71. Sexual harassment is common on college campuses.   1 2 3 4

72. If I discovered I had a sexually transmitted disease, I would tell my partner immediately.   1 2 3 4

73. If my partner or I were sterile, I would seek some form of reproductive engineering to have a child as "naturally" as possible.   1 2 3 4

74. An exhibitionist is a nuisance, not a criminal.   1 2 3 4

75. The male and female reproductive systems are more similar than different.   1 2 3 4

76. Drinking on a date allows me to relax and enjoy myself more.   1 2 3 4

77. If I were pregnant or got my girlfriend pregnant, I would tell my parents.   1 2 3 4

78. Young people should be allowed to behave more or less as they please regarding sexual matters.   1 2 3 4

79. Whenever I meet someone new that I like, I get nervous and don't know what to say.   1 2 3 4

80. Sometimes I am forced to go out on a date by a friend when I really don't want to.   1 2 3 4

81. Through the eyes of the person we love, we see ourselves in a very positive way.   1 2 3 4

82. Loneliness appears to be the major negative aspect of living alone.   1 2 3 4

83. Love justifies sex.   1 2 3 4

84. I would use a computer dating service or place an ad in the newspaper for a date.   1 2 3 4

85. The major conflicts my partner and I have are about our friends, money, and sex.   1 2 3 4

Reviewing Important Concepts

1. Defend the statement "We are all sexual beings."

2. How do biological, psychological, and cultural factors influence our sexuality? Which is the most important and why?

3. How does a positive sexual self-concept influence your self-esteem? Can your self-esteem enhance your feelings of sexual adequacy? How?

4. Identify three ways in which a human sexuality course can improve sexual communication.

5. Three destructive elements in a relationship are exploitation, excessive dependency, and jealousy. Define each of these terms and explain why each is potentially destructive to a healthy relationship.

Self-Discovery

1. Your parents have just discovered your human sexuality textbook, complete with its illustrations. Explain to them why you are taking a human sexuality course.

2. Describe your current sexual self-concept. Does it allow you to form intimate relationships with others? Why or why not?

3. Recall the sources and content of your own sex education. At what age should human sexuality first be taught? Identify the content of this course.

4. As a college student, what do you expect to learn from a human sexuality course? How would the expectations of men and women differ? Why?

5. Describe those acceptable and unacceptable sexual behaviors that our culture has adopted. Which ones do you disagree with and why?

6. What sexual values or ethics do you feel should be included in a course on human sexuality? Which should be excluded and why?

7. How has your own religious background influenced your views on sexuality and your behavior?

8. Are you satisfied with your close relationships to family members and friends? Why or why not? How could this course improve those relationships?

9. In your opinion, is the recent trend toward greater acceptance of sexuality likely to continue? Why or why not?

10. Do you feel it is possible for a human sexuality course to lower the incidence of sexually transmitted diseases in the United States? Why or why not?

Self-Quizzes

How well do you know this material? Test yourself by answering the following sample questions.

True/False

_____ 1. The primary reason for studying human sexuality is to improve sexual communication.

_____ 2. Sexual exploitation involves using someone to our sexual advantage.

_____ 3. Self-esteem influences our sexual feelings and behavior.

_____ 4. Inaccurate information about sex can sometimes lead to sexual problems.

_____ 5. People with physical disabilities, people who are mentally retarded, and older people are not sexual beings.

_____ 6. It is believed that the human brain undergoes sexual differentiation prior to birth.

_____ 7. Self-fulfilling prophecies are expectations that influence our behavior in such ways that our expectations are fulfilled.

_____ 8. Masturbation is not acceptable in our cultural milieu.

_____ 9. Sexual research reported in the media needs to be carefully analyzed for inaccuracies.

_____ 10. The sexual ethics of the teacher is the most important determinant of a quality human sexuality course.

Matching

_____ 1. Gender identity   A. Having only one spouse at a time
_____ 2. Jealousy   B. Whether one is male or female based on his or her genitalia
_____ 3. Monogamy   C. Sex involving a close relative
_____ 4. Sex   D. Excessive dependency
_____ 5. Incest   E. Whether one psychologically feels oneself to be male or to be female

Answer Key to Self-Quizzes

True/False

1. F	6. T
2. T	7. T
3. T	8. F
4. T	9. T
5. F	10. F

Matching

1. E
2. D
3. A
4. B
5. C

2 Judging Sexual Research

Sexology (the scientific study of sex) is an exciting young field that has developed over the past century. Although we have learned much regarding sexual behavior during that time, sexual research is still in its infancy stage. Virtually every newspaper, magazine, and television newscast includes some sexual revelation daily. However, how can we separate sense from nonsense, research-based facts from personal opinion? Designing, conducting, and interpreting research findings is no easy task. Let's see how well *you* can do as a sexual researcher in the following situations.

Investigation 1

The following questions regarding sexual activity provide little information to the researcher, may close off a sensitive area with a yes/no response, or cannot be objectively measured. Rewrite each of the questions into a researchable question so that you can obtain important information about human sexual attitudes and behaviors. Three examples are given to help you in this endeavor, with the first question in each being incorrect and the second question rewritten as a research question.

Example A: Have you ever had intercourse?
            At about what age did you first have intercourse?
Example B: Do you use contraceptives?
            What type of contraceptives do you use?
Example C: Have you ever had a sexually transmitted disease?
            Which sexually transmitted diseases have you been exposed to?

1. Have you ever experienced multiple orgasms?

2. Is premarital sexual intercourse wrong?

3. Does a person masturbate when he or she is unhappy with his or her marriage?

4. Should sex education start in kindergarten?

5. When pornography is shown to men, does it lead to sexual assault?

6. Is teenage pregnancy the result of poverty?

7. Should research be permitted on frozen embryos?

8. Is surrogate motherhood immoral?

9. When two individuals with mental handicaps marry each other, does it spread mental retardation?

10. Have you ever engaged in oral sex?

Investigation 2

Using the research questions from Investigation 1, select one item and design a research study to answer that question. Be sure to include the following information:

1. Design (data collection procedure)
   a. case studies
   b. experimental research
   c. observational research
   d. survey research
2. Sample selection procedure and size
3. Description of sample participants (age, gender, economic status, educational level, religion)
4. Informed consent procedure
5. Data analysis
6. Limitations of the study (where or how the sample was drawn, number of nonrespondents)

Investigation 3

After reading the following two studies, indicate the error that has occurred in the conclusions.

1. A team of doctors visited mental institutions in eight western states. After careful observation, the team noted that patients spent a lot of time masturbating. It was concluded that masturbation causes mental illness.

2. An intern working at the Centers for Disease Control received health information from ten local clinics indicating that eighteen new cases of tuberculosis were diagnosed in female prostitutes. The intern quickly issued a bulletin stating that tuberculosis was linked to hypersexuality.

Reviewing Important Concepts

1. Explain the advantages and limitations of case studies, experimental research, observational research, and survey research.

2. Why will the results of a study be biased if the sample is not randomly selected?

3. What is a double-blind study? Is this method applicable to all research studies? Why or why not?

4. What is the relationship between validity and reliability? Is one more important than the other? Why or why not?

5. Compare and contrast descriptive and analytical studies. Which could be generalized to a wider population and why?

6. Why is Alfred Kinsey's research still respected and referred to today?

7. How did William Masters and Virginia Johnson approach the study of human sexuality? What impact did their research have on sex therapy?

8. Describe the characteristics of ethical sexual research.

9. What can be done to minimize the negative effects of sexual research on the participant or on his or her relationships?

10. Compare and contrast the quality of sexual research in the popular media and professional publications.

Self-Discovery

1. How might your own personal biases influence your methodology or the interpretation of your research results?

2. If you were involved in a sex survey, would you be more likely to exaggerate or minimize your sexual experiences? Why?

3. Do you feel that you could predict the answers to a sex survey if you knew the respondents' age, gender, educational level, religious beliefs, economic level, political beliefs, or geographic location? Why or why not?

4. Do you agree with the statement "Scientific research is ethically neutral; it merely describes, predicts, and explains"? Why or why not?

5. You and your roommate are both asked to participate in a sexuality research study. Your roommate quickly volunteers. What factors would affect your decision to participate? If you reluctantly agreed to participate, how would this affect the results of the study?

6. Do you feel that a researcher is obligated to explain to a participant the possible positive and negative side effects of a study? Should every participant be required to give his or her written consent? Explain.

7. Should researchers be given more freedom to investigate sexual topics, problems, or populations? Why or why not?

Self-Quizzes

How well do you know this material? Test yourself by answering the following sample questions.

True/False

_____ 1. Sex research is dependent upon volunteers, a fact that does not affect the results.

_____ 2. A control group is a group of subjects who receive no treatment.

_____ 3. Most of our scientific knowledge of human sexuality has come from experimental research using a double-blind technique.

_____ 4. Case studies focus in depth on particular individuals.

_____ 5. The results of a sex study are less reliable as the sample size increases because of the wide variation within the population.

_____ 6. The greatest advantage of magazine surveys is the large number of respondents, even though they may not be a representative cross section of the U.S. population.

_____ 7. Sexuality material published in such magazines as *Discover, Newsweek,* and *Redbook* would be reliable.

_____ 8. One of the major disadvantages of surveys is that people tend to underreport undesirable information.

_____ 9. In order to ensure confidentiality in a sexual research study, code numbers should be assigned to participants.

_____ 10. When a participant has been given all of the information about a study, both the positive and potential negative effects, and freely chooses to become involved in the study, then he or she has given informed consent.

_____ 11. It is possible to predict the direction of sexuality research in the future.

_____ 12. Freud theorized that the unconscious part of the mind can interfere with adult sexual and nonsexual functioning.

_____ 13. Clinical research has been criticized for studying only people who can afford treatment.

_____ 14. Little sexual research is done in academic settings—colleges and universities.

_____ 15. A researcher's own culture, religion, and research expectations may positively or negatively affect the collection of data in a study.

Multiple Choice

1. Which of the following individual(s) is (are) most closely associated with the case study method?
   a. Sigmund Freud
   b. Alfred Kinsey
   c. Havelock Ellis
   d. Masters and Johnson

2. Which of the following techniques would be most appropriate for assessing the sexual activity level of students on a large college campus?
   a. case study
   b. survey
   c. laboratory observation
   d. field observation

3. Most of what we know about the physiology of sexual response comes from the research of which of the following people?
   a. Shere Hite
   b. Alfred Kinsey
   c. Bell and Weinberg
   d. Masters and Johnson

4. Which of the following was the major criticism associated with Shere Hite's studies?
   a. Her sample did not represent a true cross section of the population.
   b. She used a written survey rather than an oral interview.
   c. She relied on a small sample size, which adversely affected the validity of the studies.
   d. She focused on people's feelings rather than their sexual behavior.

5. Which of the following numbers is closest to the number of participants Kinsey interviewed during his research on human sexuality?
   a. 17
   b. 170
   c. 1,700
   d. 17,000

Answer Key to Self-Quizzes

True/False

1. F	6. T	11. F
2. T	7. F	12. T
3. F	8. T	13. F
4. T	9. T	14. F
5. F	10. T	15. T

Multiple Choice

1. C
2. B
3. D
4. A
5. D

3 Values and Sexual Behavior

Sexual moral values relate to the rightness and wrongness of sexual conduct and when and how sexuality should be expressed. As our experiences change, our values evolve and mature. Therefore, our values are in a state of constant change.

Sexual Decision Making

How do you feel about each of the following behaviors or practices right now? Identify where each behavior or practice fits on the continuum line, and write the number for that behavior above that point on the line.

-------------------- X -------------------- -- -------------------- X --------------------

Acceptable to me   **Unacceptable to me**

1. Premarital sex
2. Prostitution
3. Surrogate mothers
4. Group sex
5. Sexual intercourse
6. Kissing a member of the same sex
7. Divorce
8. Sex without love
9. Oral sex
10. Heterosexual marriage

11. Masturbation to orgasm
12. Rape
13. Artificial insemination
14. French kissing
15. Genital touching
16. Anal intercourse
17. Homosexuality
18. Cohabitation
19. Polygamy
20. Abortion for myself or partner

21. Homosexual marriage
22. Pornography
23. In vitro fertilization
24. Bisexuality
25. Sterilization
26. Adultery
27. Interracial sex
28. Love without sex
29. Petting
30. Sexual double standard for men and women

Kidney Dialysis Dilemma

You are the chairman of the hospital review board in your community. Four people are in desperate need of the one and only kidney dialysis machine in your hospital, but only one person can be accommodated. Each person will die in two months if he or she does not begin dialysis immediately. The four patients are (a) a lesbian, (b) a gay male, (c) a prostitute, and (d) a male transsexual.

1. To whom do you offer the dialysis treatment?

2. How do you decide which person shall receive treatment and live?

3. How would you feel if you found out that the three people who died would have found a cure for AIDS, cancer, and heart disease if they had lived?

Reviewing Important Concepts

1. Describe three positive and three negative reasons why people engage in sexual activity.

2. Do you agree with the statement "It is important that we consciously and deliberately script all of our sexual behavior in terms of our sexual values"? Why or why not?

3. How does scripting limit our choice in a sexual partner?

4. Compare and contrast Kohlberg's three levels of moral reasoning. At what level are most of your friends? Why? If your friends were asked at what level *you* are, what would they say? Why?

5. Are guilty feelings based on our values, or do our values develop because of guilty feelings?

6. What is the difference between value indicators and value criteria? Give an example of each.

7. Compare and contrast the position of women in the Hebrew, Greek, and Roman civilizations. Describe the sexual double standard that men were allowed in these societies.

8. How did the rise of the Reformation change attitudes toward sex? Briefly describe the impact of Martin Luther and John Calvin on marriage.

9. Have developments in science and technology positively or negatively affected our sexual values? Give an example of a development in each area and explain its effect.

10. Lewis Smedes identifies three basic moral questions as the basis for sexual decision-making. Briefly explain each. What might be the fourth question that a deeply religious person would ask?

Self-Discovery

1. How have your values changed in the past five years?

2. Do you feel your partner could influence you to change your views on premarital sex? If so, how?

3. What sexual values do you adhere to that you believe cannot be changed or influenced by others? Why?

4. When evaluating your sexual values in any given situation, do you make your decisions on the basis of what is best for you or best for your partner? Explain.

5. Was your first sexual experience a free choice out of love for your partner or pressure from your partner? Explain.

6. What values must be met before you would consider sleeping with your partner?

7. Under what circumstances would you have a relationship with a married person?

8. What would you do if your partner's best friend made sexual advances toward you?

9. When you are in a committed relationship with someone, why would you choose not to publicly affirm it?

10. Just because you feel a sexual attraction for someone, does that in itself give you the right to pursue a relationship? Why or why not?

Self-Quizzes

How well do you know this material? Test yourself by answering the following sample questions.

Fill in the Blanks

1. Those values that deal with a person's conduct and treatment of other people are called _____ .

2. Values that relate to when and how sexuality should be expressed are called _____ values.

3. Besides parents, the most influential source of sexual information is _____ .

4. According to Gagnon, sexual _____ determine the who, what, when, where, and why of our sexual behavior.

5. A goal is a(n) _____ that indicates an intended course of action that may or may not be completed.

6. In order to control population, both the Greeks and the Romans practiced abortion and _____ , especially during times of food shortages.

7. Greek women who provided entertainment and sexual gratification were referred to as _____ .

8. According to Plato and Aristotle, the highest form of human friendship was possible only between _____ .

9. In the _____ culture, if a man died without having any children, it became his brother's duty to marry and impregnate the widow.

10. The semen theory was a pivotal theme in _____ values.

Matching

_____ 1. Viewed semen as a vital substance essential to a man's well-being and health

_____ 2. Level of moral reasoning based upon an internal, self-defined, set of beliefs and values

_____ 3. An early follower of Christ who saw sexual intercourse as uniting two people—body and soul—to each other

_____ 4. A Roman Catholic bishop who had been married, fathered a child, and associated guilt rather than pleasure with sex

_____ 5. Condemned fornication because of the possible adverse effects upon the child conceived out of wedlock

_____ 6. Viewed marriage as both a religious and a civic affair

_____ 7. Actions that adversely affect a person's self-worth and the realization of his or her full potential

_____ 8. The ideology with which the statement "Whatever is the most loving thing in the situation is the right and good thing" is associated

_____ 9. Sexual behavior that Jesus condemned for men and women

_____ 10. Advocated strict dress codes aimed at limiting stimulation of the senses, but considered sex within marriage natural and good

A. Martin Luther
B. St. Thomas Aquinas
C. Situational morality
D. St. Paul
E. Postconventional morality
F. Immoral actions
G. Victorians
H. St. Augustine
I. Adultery
J. Conventional morality
K. Homosexuality
L. Traditional morality
M. Puritans
N. John Calvin

Answer Key to Self-Quizzes

Fill in the Blanks

1. moral	6. infanticide
2. sexual	7. pornae
3. peers	8. men
4. scripts	9. Hebrew
5. value indicator	10. Victorian

Matching

1. G	6. A
2. E	7. F
3. D	8. C
4. H	9. I
5. B	10. M

4 Love and Intimacy

I love pizza! I love my dog! I love my mother! Since the beginning of time, man has tried to define the word *love*. To each of us, it has many different meanings. Kahlil Gibran, a noted philosopher and poet, wrote the following about love:

The Prophet

When love beckons to you, follow him,
Though his ways are hard and steep.
And when his wings enfold you yield to him,
Though the sword hidden among his pinions may wound you.
And when he speaks to you believe in him,
Though his voice may shatter your dreams as the north wind lays waste the garden.

For even as love crowns you so shall he crucify you. Even as he is for your growth so is he for your pruning.
Even as he ascends to your height and caresses your tenderest branches that quiver in the sun,
So shall he descend to your roots and shake them in their clinging to the earth. . . .

But if in your fear you would seek only love's peace and love's pleasure,
Then it is better for you that you cover your nakedness and pass out of love's threshing-floor,
Into the seasonless world where you shall laugh, but not all of your laughter, and weep, but not all of your tears.

Love gives naught but itself and takes naught but from itself.
Love possesses not nor would it be possessed;
For love is sufficient unto love.

When you love you should not say, "God is in my heart," but rather, "I am in the heart of God."
And think not you can direct the course of love, for love, if it finds you worthy, directs your course.

Reprinted from *The Prophet,* by Kahlil Gibran, by permission of Alfred A. Knopf, Inc. Copyright 1923 by Kahlil Gibran and renewed 1951 by Administrators C.T.A. of Kahlil Gibran Estate and Mary G. Gibran.

1. Do you agree with Gibran's description of love? Why or why not?

2. What section(s) of this poem is (are) the most meaningful to you? Why?

3. Which part of this poem would your mother say is the most meaningful to her? Your father?

What Love Means to Me

On the basis of your own experiences, circle the ten words or phrases that best define what love means to you *now*. Put an X by the five words or phrases that you would never associate with love. Finally, put two stars by the words or phrases that you think will describe love for you five years from now.

Physical attractiveness	A sense of humor
Self-confidence	Togetherness
Compromise	Trust
Jealousy	Respect
Loyalty	Open communication
Emotional intimacy	Faithfulness
Tenderness	Empathy
Sacrifice	Forgiveness
Marriage	Understanding
Security	Possessiveness
Kindness	Sharing
Never having to say I'm sorry	Expressing my emotions openly
Honesty	Commitment
Caring about my physical appearance	Putting my partner's needs before my own
Independence	Dependence
Warm fuzzies	Friendship
Children	Unconditional acceptance
Compassion	Caring
Physical intimacy	Being able to take out my frustrations
Being there when I need them	Obsessiveness
Responsibility	Privacy
Freedom	Self-disclosure
Vulnerability	

1. Did any of your answers surprise you? Why or why not?

2. How did your answers change when you projected yourself five years into the future?

I Know That My Partner Loves Me Because He or She . . .

Using the list below, rate the five most important statements that describe a loving relationship (rank these in order from 1 through 5).

a. makes me feel important whether we are alone together or in a crowd of a thousand
b. satisfies my physical needs
c. satisfies my emotional needs
d. satisfies both my physical and emotional needs
e. never makes me suspicious or jealous
f. is always someone I can depend on to be concerned about my happiness
g. is always surprising me with reminders of his or her affection

h. allows me to be myself and feel independent while united to him or her
i. listens when I need to expound
j. offers nonjudgmental thoughts in problem solving
k. accepts me unconditionally
l. keeps our relationship the number 1 priority in his or her life
m. is willing to express his or her innermost feelings
n. allows me some private time for myself
o. always calls and lets me know when he or she is delayed
p. treats me with gentleness and tenderness

Reviewing Important Concepts

1. What is the difference between emotional intimacy and sexual intimacy? Why does a relationship disintegrate if emotional intimacy is missing?

2. In his classic *Why Am I Afraid to Tell You Who I Am?*, John Powell identifies five rules for self-disclosure. Identify and explain these rules for gut-level communication.

3. Compare and contrast the behavioral, psychoanalytic, and humanistic views of love. Which do you agree with and why?

4. How and why may love be viewed as an "addiction"?

5. How may low levels of jealousy actually enhance a relationship? Why might a person try to make his or her partner jealous?

6. Explain the differences between self-love, conceit, and lack of consideration of others.

Self-Discovery

1. If you were going to advertise yourself as a lover, what qualities would you identify?

2. Growth and change are an important part of maintaining a relationship. What kinds of things are you willing to do to maintain the vitality in your intimate relationships?

3. The goal of every person is to develop a positive self-concept, which includes independence and self-reliance. An even greater goal for most people is emotional intimacy, which involves a deep commitment to someone else. How can you strike a balance between these two concepts—personal identity and intimacy?

4. Which should you listen to in a love relationship: your head or your heart? Why?

5. If you are attracted to someone, are you hesitant to reveal your affections until you are sure the feelings are mutual? Why or why not?

Self-Quizzes

How well do you know this material? Test yourself by answering the following sample questions.

True/False

_____ 1. The "halo" effect says that physically attractive people are assumed to possess more desirable characteristics than average-looking people.

_____ 2. How a person looks is more important to older people than to younger people.

_____ 3. As the old adage says, "opposites attract."

_____ 4. Humanists typically study emotionally healthy people rather than people with problems.

_____ 5. Intimacy can only develop when we are willing to reveal our innermost feelings to another person.

_____ 6. Jealousy occurs when we are secure about ourselves and our relationship.

_____ 7. Most people "fall in love" rapidly and suddenly but "fall out of love" very slowly.

_____ 8. The most common cause of the inability to love is low self-esteem.

_____ 9. An excessively dependent partner is likely to be perceived as selfish.

_____ 10. Behaviorists view love as a learned response, based on rewarding or reinforcing experiences.

_____ 11. Liking is simply a lesser degree of loving someone.

___ 12. The amount of commitment we bring to a relationship is dependent upon whether or not our parents have been divorced.

___ 13. Sex with affection is more rewarding than sex without love.

___ 14. The first step in "falling out of love" is realizing that your "ex" is unworthy of your love.

___ 15. Intimacy is a holistic concept that includes emotional, intellectual, social, and spiritual bonds.

Multiple Choice

1. According to Fromm, which of the following characteristics is *not* necessary for love?
   a. responsibility
   b. trust
   c. respect
   d. physical attractiveness

2. Which of the following theories states that partners do not necessarily fulfill the same needs for each other, but feel they are giving and receiving about equally?
   a. exchange theory
   b. equity theory
   c. reinforcement theory
   d. wheel theory

3. Which of the following statements would be associated with Sigmund Freud?
   a. Love of self and love of others is incompatible.
   b. People become human through loving.
   c. Love is an equal caring and giving process.
   d. Love is the primary human motivating force.

4. Which of the following is a state that involves friendly affection and a deep attachment to another person?
   a. limerance
   b. passionate love
   c. companionate love
   d. infatuation

5. Effective communication requires all of the following *except*
   a. being an active listener.
   b. using "you" statements.
   c. making sure you have plenty of time for your discussion.
   d. being alert to body language.

Answer Key to Self-Quizzes

True/False

1. T	6. F	11. F
2. F	7. F	12. F
3. F	8. T	13. T
4. T	9. F	14. F
5. T	10. T	15. T

Multiple Choice

1. D
2. B
3. A
4. C
5. B

5 Male Sexual Anatomy and Physiology

Many of us know relatively little about our own reproductive system or that of the other sex. In addition, we often have preconceived ideas about what it means to be male or female. Would you want to be a male today?

Thoughts on Being Male

Complete the following questionnaire by indicating the degree to which you agree or disagree with each of the statements, using the scale below. There are no correct or incorrect responses to these statements.

Strongly Agree	Agree	Disagree	Strongly Disagree
1	2	3	4

1. It is important for males to perform a self-testicular exam in order to prevent testicular cancer.   1 2 3 4

2. Most men would be better lovers if they spent more time on foreplay.   1 2 3 4

3. Men have a more romantic view of relationships than do women.   1 2 3 4

4. During self-disclosure, men are more likely to reveal their strengths and not mention their weaknesses.   1 2 3 4

5. Most men are afraid to touch another man.   1 2 3 4

6. Children need fathers to take a more active role in child rearing.   1 2 3 4

7. College men are more willing to cohabitate than college women.   1 2 3 4

8. A man is more embarrassed when he is examined by a female doctor than a woman is when she is examined by a male doctor.   1 2 3 4

9. Homosexual males have more partners than heterosexual males because they do not have the stability of marriage.   1 2 3 4

10. Every man experiences impotence at some time in his life.   1 2 3 4

11. After a massive heart attack, men should refrain from sexual intercourse.   1 2 3 4

12. A physically fit male is more sexually attractive than an unfit male.   1 2 3 4

13. An effective birth control pill should be developed for use by the male.   1 2 3 4

14. If a woman is pregnant, she should obtain permission from the man who impregnated her before she may have an abortion.   1 2 3 4

15. It is an undue financial hardship for men to pay alimony.   1 2 3 4

16. All men should be circumcised at birth.   1 2 3 4

17. Most men can express anger more easily than most women.   1 2 3 4

18. Fetal alcohol syndrome may be caused by the father's drinking patterns as well as the mother's.   1 2 3 4

19. The traditional male script focuses on sex over feelings.   1 2 3 4

20. It is the male's responsibility to be the breadwinner for the family.   1 2 3 4

21. For men, *how* they are touched is more important to them than it is to women.   1 2 3 4

22. Men have a larger, more varied sexual vocabulary than women.   1 2 3 4

23. Men communicate more nonverbally than women.   1 2 3 4

24. If a couple decides not to have any more children, then the man should have a vasectomy.   1 2 3 4

25. The majority of condoms are purchased by women.   1 2 3 4

Reviewing Important Concepts

1. In what ways are penile erection and vaginal lubrication similar?

2. Describe a testicular self-examination.

3. Briefly explain the vascular processes in penile erection.

4. Explain why it is not possible for a boy to ejaculate before he has reached puberty.

5. Describe the two stages of ejaculation. What is emission, and when does it occur?

6. Define hormone, target tissues, and receptor sites.

7. How does the "negative feedback loop" function to keep testosterone levels fairly constant?

8. Describe the hypothalamus-pituitary-testes "connection." Which hormones are released from which source? What effect does each hormone have? What mechanism controls this process?

9. Why does the sperm count have to be so high for the male to be considered fertile? What change in sperm needs to occur for an egg to be fertilized?

10. Explain the relationship between testosterone level and sexual desire and how it differs in males and females.

Self-Discovery

1. Describe puberty and the male anatomy to your eight-year-old son.

2. Would you feel uncomfortable if your partner asked *you* to perform his self-testicular or her breast exam? Why or why not?

3. Describe a conversation between high school girls in a locker room talking about male anatomy. Would women in a health club locker room discuss the same topics and have the same attitudes? Explain.

4. Your doctor asks you whether or not you would like your newborn son circumcised. What would influence your decision?

5. How would a teenage girl describe the physiological aspect of a male erection? How would this differ from a teenage boy's description of the same process?

6. **If you are male . . .**

   a. How did you feel the first time you shaved your face? How old were you? Were you older or younger than your friends?

   b. What part(s) of your anatomy are you uncomfortable with? Why?

   c. What do you believe has contributed to your negative feelings?

   d. Are you uncomfortable to the degree that it inhibits your sexuality with your partner? If so, what can you do to change your feelings toward your body?

   e. What in particular do you want your partner to know about your anatomy?

Self-Quizzes

How well do you know this material? Test yourself by answering the following sample questions.

True/False

___ 1. A male must have an erection in order to ejaculate.

___ 2. Sperm are produced in the seminiferous tubules and mature in the epididymis.

___ 3. The penis has a bone in it that can be felt when the penis is erect.

___ 4. Testosterone is responsible for sexual desire in males.

___ 5. The temperature of the testes is three to four degrees Fahrenheit cooler than normal body temperature.

___ 6. There is evidence that penis size is important in giving a woman sexual pleasure.

___ 7. The external sex organs consist of the penis, testes, and scrotum.

___ 8. The corpora cavernosa and corpus spongiosum are found in the penis.

___ 9. The life expectancy of a sperm cell is twenty-four to thirty-six hours.

___ 10. The head of a sperm cell contains the chromosomal material.

___ 11. Ejaculation in a boy is not possible until he has reached puberty.

___ 12. Secretions from the prostate gland make up about 70 percent of the total volume of semen.

___ 13. Sperm leave the testes via the vas deferens.

___ 14. The seminal vesicles are the sites of sperm storage and maturation.

___ 15. Circumcision is surgical removal of the corona.

___ 16. The prostate gland is located directly beneath the bladder.

___ 17. Fluid from the Cowper's gland neutralizes the acidity of the urethra.

___ 18. Hormones are chemical substances produced and secreted by endocrine glands.

___ 19. Interstitial cell-stimulating hormone (ICSH) is chemically identical to luteinizing hormone (LH) in the female.

___ 20. Sertoli cells release the hormone oxytocin.

___ 21. The pituitary gland is the primary controlling mechanism in the male reproductive system.

___ 22. It is possible for a woman to become pregnant even if the penis is withdrawn prior to ejaculation.

___ 23. Sperm motility is aided by prostaglandins secreted from the seminal vesicles.

___ 24. The Cowper's glands are doughnut-shaped and surround the urethra.

___ 25. Undescended testes produce a condition known as an inguinal hernia.

Identification: Male Sex Organs

Label the diagram with the correct terms.

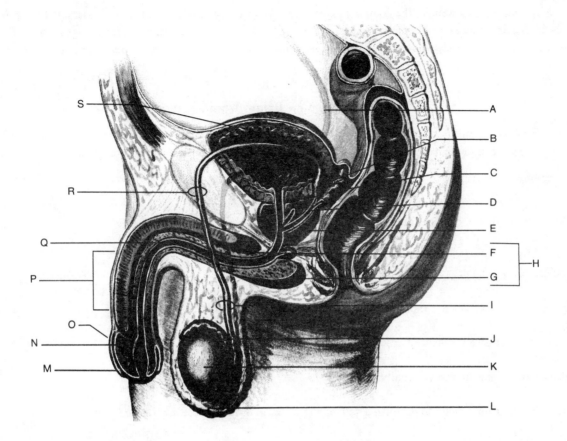

Figure 5.1 Male Sex Organs

From John W. Hole, Jr., *Human Anatomy and Physiology*, 5th ed. Copyright © 1990 Wm. C. Brown Publishers, Dubuque, Iowa. All Rights Reserved. Reprinted by permission.

Answer Key to Self-Quizzes

True/False

1. F	6. F	11. T	16. T	21. F
2. T	7. F	12. F	17. T	22. T
3. F	8. T	13. T	18. T	23. T
4. T	9. F	14. F	19. T	24. F
5. T	10. T	15. F	20. F	25. F

Identification: Male Sex Organs

A. Ureter
B. Ampulla
C. Seminal vesicle
D. Ejaculatory duct
E. Prostate gland
F. Crus
G. Bulb
H. Base of penis
I. Vas deferens
J. Epididymis

K. Testis
L. Scrotum
M. Prepuce
N. Glans
O. Coronal ridge
P. Penis
Q. Urethra
R. Vas deferens
S. Urinary bladder

6 Female Sexual Anatomy and Physiology

Before you are able to comprehend the complex psychological aspects of sexual functioning, you must have a basic knowledge of the anatomy and physiology of the female body. However, let's examine your feelings on what it means to be female in a predominantly male society. Based on *your* answers, would you want to be a female in today's society?

Thoughts on Being Female

Complete the following questionnaire by indicating the degree to which you agree or disagree with each of the statements, using the scale below. There are no correct or incorrect responses to these statements.

Strongly Agree	Agree	Disagree	Strongly Disagree
1	2	3	4

1. The woman's movement has raised the consciousness of both men and women about the need for sexual equality. 1 2 3 4

2. The intensity of an orgasm in a female is greater than an orgasm in a male. 1 2 3 4

3. Large-breasted women are more sexually attractive than small-breasted women. 1 2 3 4

4. Sexually aggressive women are described by men as adventurous. 1 2 3 4

5. Women communicate more verbally than men. 1 2 3 4

6. It is important for women to perform a self-breast exam in order to detect breast cancer. 1 2 3 4

7. During self-disclosure, women are more likely to reveal their weaknesses and not mention their strengths. 1 2 3 4

8. Most women have a very close female friend whom they can talk to about any sexual problem. 1 2 3 4

9. Women are more likely to pick up an attractive, young male hitchhiker than an older man. 1 2 3 4

10. If a man father's a child, he should pay child support until the child graduates from college or is twenty-one years old. 1 2 3 4

11. The traditional female script focuses on caring over physical intimacy. 1 2 3 4

12. For women, *where* they are touched is more important to them than it is to men. 1 2 3 4

13. Lesbians living in a monogamous relationship would like to legally marry each other. 1 2 3 4

14. Most women would be better lovers if they spent more time on manual stimulation. 1 2 3 4

15. It is the woman's responsibility to be the care giver for the children. 1 2 3 4

16. A woman is more embarrassed buying condoms than a man is buying tampax. 1 2 3 4

17. In general, women are much less hesitant than men to involve themselves in a new relationship. 1 2 3 4

18. If a woman returns a man's smile, he can be reasonably sure that she is sexually interested in him. 1 2 3 4

19. Today, more women than men tell "off-color" jokes. 1 2 3 4

20. Divorced females have a more difficult time finding a date than do divorced males. 1 2 3 4

21. If a woman is still a virgin in today's society, she is considered a "cold fish." 1 2 3 4

22. In reality, only a few women are multiorgasmic. 1 2 3 4

23. Most men and women have some type of sexual fantasy every day. 1 2 3 4

24. If a wife's salary is greater than her husband's, his masculinity is threatened. 1 2 3 4

25. The ultimate responsibility of birth control is the woman's, as she is the one who gets pregnant. 1 2 3 4

Reviewing Important Concepts

1. The vagina is considered to be the organ of intercourse for the female. What are three additional functions of the vagina?

2. Identify five factors that contribute to the development of vaginal infections.

3. Briefly describe a gynecological exam. What is the purpose of a Pap smear?

4. What are the symptoms of toxic shock syndrome? How can it be prevented?

5. Identify the secondary sex characteristics that are associated with estrogen secretions.

6. What two gonadotropins are present in both the male and the female?

7. What are some of the physical, emotional, and behavioral symptoms of PMS (premenstrual syndrome)?

8. What is believed to be the cause of dysmenorrhea? How can it be treated?

9. What health benefits are associated with breast-feeding?

10. Briefly describe the effects the following hormones have on lactation: insulin, estrogen, progesterone, prolactin, prolactin-inhibiting hormone, and oxytocin.

Self-Discovery

1. Describe the menstrual cycle to your eight-year-old daughter.

2. Would you engage in sexual activity with your partner while you are (she is) menstruating? Why or why not?

3. Would you feel uncomfortable if your partner asked *you* to perform her breast exam or his testicular exam? Why or why not?

4. Reflecting upon the female genitalia and anatomy, what preferences do you have (i.e., large breasts)? What characteristics do you not prefer?

5. Describe a conversation between high school boys in a locker room talking about female anatomy. Would men in a health club locker room discuss the same topics and have the same attitudes? Explain.

Self-Quizzes

How well do you know this material? Test yourself by answering the following sample questions.

True/False

_____ 1. The breasts are considered part of the external genitalia.

_____ 2. The vaginal opening is partially covered by a membrane called the perineum.

_____ 3. The endometrium is the inner layer of the uterus.

_____ 4. The clitoris is analogous to the penis.

_____ 5. Cystitis is the name given to a condition in which endometrial tissue, normally found in the uterus, grows in other places.

_____ 6. At birth, a female has the maximum number of ova she will ever have, approximately 34,000.

_____ 7. Estrogen and progesterone are secreted by the ovaries.

_____ 8. A Pap smear can detect ovarian cancer.

_____ 9. Eighty percent of the cases of toxic shock syndrome occur in women under age thirty.

_____ 10. Progesterone treatment for premenstrual syndrome is highly controversial because of its many side effects.

_____ 11. Breast self-examination should be done monthly, at the beginning of the menstrual flow.

_____ 12. High levels of androgens are associated with a high sex drive in women.

_____ 13. Fertilization normally occurs in the fallopian tubes.

_____ 14. Ovulation occurs approximately fourteen days before the next menstrual cycle begins.

_____ 15. Human chorionic gonadotropin is only present when a woman is breast-feeding.

_____ 16. Each menstrual cycle begins when the hypothalamus secretes GnRF, which in turn stimulates the pituitary gland to secrete FSH and LH.

_____ 17. Variations in the size of a woman's breast are due to the amount of milk-producing glandular tissue present.

_____ 18. Amenorrhea is painful or difficult menstruation.

_____ 19. Vaginal lubrication results from the secretions of the Bartholin glands.

_____ 20. Orgasm, with or without a partner, helps relieve menstrual cramps.

_____ 21. The vulva is defined as the external female genitalia.

_____ 22. Milk secretion by the breasts is stimulated by the hormone oxytocin.

_____ 23. A diet high in sugar is associated with vaginitis.

_____ 24. The area between the labia minora that contains the vaginal and urethral openings is called the vestibule.

_____ 25. The upper third of the uterus is called the areola.

Identification: Female Sex Organs

Label the diagrams with the correct terms.

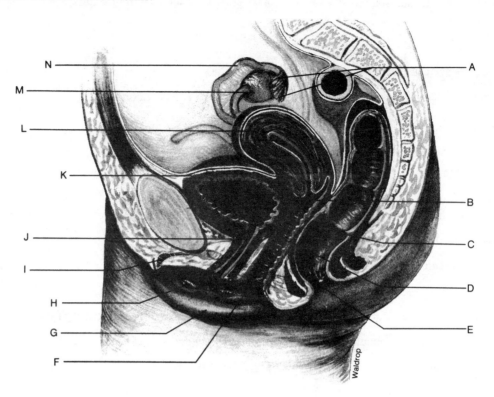

Figure 6.1 Female Internal Sex Organs

From John W. Hole, Jr., *Human Anatomy and Physiology*, 5th ed. Copyright © 1990 Wm. C. Brown Publishers, Dubuque, Iowa. All Rights Reserved. Reprinted by permission.

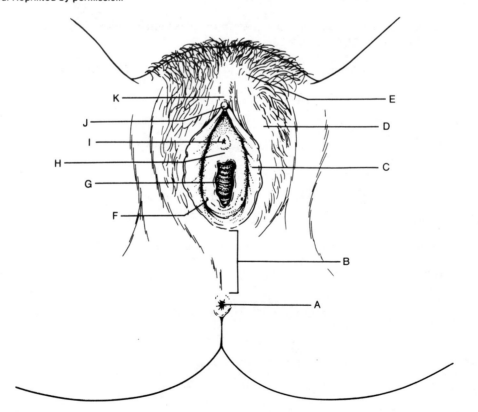

Figure 6.2 Female External Sex Organs

From John W. Hole, Jr., *Human Anatomy and Physiology*, 5th ed. Copyright © 1990 Wm. C. Brown Publishers, Dubuque, Iowa. All Rights Reserved. Reprinted by permission.

Answer Key to Self-Quizzes

True/False

1. F	6. F	11. F	16. T	21. T
2. F	7. T	12. T	17. F	22. F
3. T	8. F	13. T	18. F	23. T
4. T	9. T	14. T	19. F	24. T
5. F	10. T	15. F	20. T	25. F

Identification: Female Sex Organs

Figure 6.1

A. Fimbrae
B. Cervix
C. Rectum
D. Vagina
E. Anus
F. Vaginal orifice
G. Labia majora
H. Labia minora
I. Clitoris
J. Urethra
K. Urinary bladder
L. Uterus
M. Ovary
N. Fallopian tube

Figure 6.2

A. Anus
B. Perineum
C. Labia minora
D. Labia majora
E. Mons veneris
F. Opening of Bartholin's glands
G. Vaginal opening
H. Vestibule
I. Urethral opening
J. Clitoris
K. Clitoral hood (prepuce)

7 Sexually Transmitted Diseases

Seldom in the history of our nation has sexual interaction, or the results thereof, captured such widespread attention as it has recently. The emotions, conflicting views, and politics of various sexual practices have been exposed. Many of us scrutinize with greater intensity than ever the end result of our sexual choices.

Research Projects

This assignment will give you the opportunity to decide how you would allocate money, time, and attention to various sexually transmitted diseases. You are the director of the Centers for Disease Control, and it is your responsibility to award large sums of money to projects that will reduce the incidence of sexually transmitted diseases. Your total budget is $200 million, and you must decide how much will be spent on each disease and how it will be divided between free clinics, education, and research. Indicate the amount of money you would assign to each STD listed below and then divide it accordingly.

	Amount of Money	Free Clinics	Education	Research
A. AIDS				
B. Genital herpes				
C. Chlamydia				
D. Gonorrhea				
E. Syphilis				
F. Candidiasis				
G. Papilloma viruses				

1. How did you decide which STD received the most money? The least money?

2. How did you decide how much of the money for each STD would be allocated to free clinics, education, and research?

Larry, MaryAnn, and Anni

At Larry's ten-year high school reunion, he meets MaryAnn, his old high school sweetheart. After several drinks and lots of reminiscing, MaryAnn invites Larry back to her apartment for a nightcap. After some more talking and laughing about the "good old days," they become intimate and have sexual intercourse. The next day, Larry goes out with his steady girlfriend, Anni, and they have intercourse that night. One week later, Larry feels a burning sensation when he urinates and notices a pus discharge from his penis. After a culture test, his doctor confirms that Larry has gonorrhea.

1. Who was the host who had gonorrhea first?

2. Who gave Larry gonorrhea? Explain your reasoning.

3. Who may Larry have given gonorrhea to and why?

4. Whom should Larry inform that he has gonorrhea? Why?

5. How would you feel if you were Larry? MaryAnn? Anni?

Reviewing Important Concepts

1. Why are accurate statistics on the incidence of a specific STD difficult to obtain?

2. How is the human immunodeficiency virus (HIV) different from other pathogens?

3. Identify four practices that may prevent the transmission of HIV.

4. Identify the early symptoms of AIDS.

5. What are the symptoms of genital herpes?

6. When is a person with herpes the most contagious and why?

7. List the factors that may trigger the recurrence of a herpes attack.

8. Identify the risks associated with childbearing and genital herpes.

9. How does oral acyclovir relieve herpes symptoms?

10. What is the current incidence of the papilloma virus (genital warts) in the United States? What disease have researchers recently associated with it and why?

11. Although there may be no early symptoms of chlamydia, what may be the symptoms in the male and female? What are the long-term effects of it if left untreated?

12. Describe the symptoms of gonorrhea in the male and female. What are the long-term effects of untreated gonorrhea in each sex?

13. Summarize the destruction that occurs to the circulatory system and nervous system when syphilis remains untreated.

14. Compare and contrast candidiasis and trichomoniasis. Which is more dangerous and why?

15. List and briefly discuss five ways that an individual can reduce the likelihood of becoming infected by an STD.

16. Identify three methods that public health agencies use to fight STDs.

Self-Discovery

1. If I contracted an STD, I *would* tell . . . , but I would *never* tell . . . Explain your answers.

2. If I were in a committed relationship, it would be hard for me to tell my partner that I had an STD because . . .

3. If a minor seeks treatment for an STD at a public health clinic, I feel that the parents *should/should not* be contacted because . . .

4. Suppose research efforts succeeded in developing effective vaccines against STDs. Would you be immunized? Would you have your children immunized? Explain.

5. How do medical, psychological, and social factors interact to *prevent* the *control* of sexually transmitted diseases?

6. Should drug abusers have legal access to sterile needles? Why or why not?

7. In your opinion, are there any occupations that an AIDS victim should be prohibited from having? If so, list them and explain why.

8. Who should be informed of the results of AIDS blood tests? Why?

9. Does society have a responsibility to AIDS victims? If so, what is it? If not, why not?

10. Should insurance companies be allowed to reject an individual who tests positive for the AIDS virus? Explain.

11. Jeff was diagnosed with AIDS nine months ago and continued to have intimate sexual relations with his wife, Marsha. She unexpectedly lost twenty pounds, has been tired, and feels weak. She went to her doctor and tested positive for the AIDS virus.

   a. Jeff and Marsha have only been married fifteen months. Can you be sure who gave AIDS to whom? Explain.

   b. Assuming that Jeff gave AIDS to Marsha, if Marsha dies, should Jeff be charged with involuntary manslaughter? Why or why not?

   c. If Marsha dies, can her family sue for wrongful death? Why or why not?

   d. Should Jeff be allowed to benefit from Marsha's death through her will? Why or why not?

Self-Quizzes

How well do you know this material? Test yourself by answering the following sample questions.

True/False

____ 1. The incubation period for STDs ranges from hours to years, but is usually a matter of weeks.

____ 2. A diet high in sugar is often associated with candidiasis.

____ 3. Urethritis is an inflammation of the urinary bladder.

____ 4. Papilloma viruses are the fastest growing, viral diseases.

____ 5. Congenital syphilis is transmitted during the late (tertiary) stage of syphilis.

____ 6. The *Neisseria gonorrhoeae* bacterium is inactivated when exposed to cold or dryness.

____ 7. Women using chemical-type contraceptives have lower rates of PID (pelvic inflammatory disease) than other sexually active women.

____ 8. Chlamydia is currently the most common STD in the United States.

____ 9. According to the law, you must inform your sexual partner if you are infected with an STD or you may be held liable for damages.

____ 10. A person's first herpes attack usually heals within two weeks.

___ 11. Hepatitis B is easily transmitted by blood and is characterized by jaundice, nausea, and abdominal pain.

___ 12. Untreated gonorrhea in the female may lead to sterility or ectopic pregnancies.

___ 13. Syphilis is less serious than gonorrhea because gonorrhea is a systemic infection.

___ 14. Trichomoniasis is a protozoan infection that causes a discharge that is usually thin and frothy.

___ 15. The symptoms associated with scabies include itching, pus-filled blisters, and discolored lines on the skin.

___ 16. It is impossible to transmit "crabs" by wearing your best friend's sweat pants.

___ 17. High-risk sexual partners include diabetics who inject insulin.

___ 18. In order to be effective in reducing STDs, a condom must be applied to an erect penis before any genital contact is made.

___ 19. Urinating before sexual contact helps to reduce the chance of pelvic inflammatory disease.

___ 20. In most states, minors may be treated for STDs without parental permission or notification.

Fill in the Blanks

1. A person who is symptom free is called _____ .

2. Cold sores are caused by herpes simplex virus type _____ .

3. Women who have PID are simultaneously treated for _____ and _____ .

4. The most common symptom of secondary syphilis is _____ .

5. One drug commonly prescribed to treat trichomoniasis is _____ .

What's Your Disease IQ?

Using the clues that are given, fill in the crossword puzzle. Do not leave a blank space between words. (Number 10 across contains a hyphen.)

Across

1. Protozoan that often causes pneumonia in AIDS victims
2. Bacterium that causes gonorrhea
3. Tiny creatures that burrow through the skin and cause intense itching
4. Abbreviation for human immunodeficiency virus
5. Pathogen associated with vaginal yeast infections
6. Abbreviation for a drug given to AIDS victims that extends their lives
7. Inflammation of the urinary bladder
8. Most prescribed drug for treating herpes
9. Another name for open sores
10. Serious viral infection of the liver

Down

11. Virus that can cause sores in the mouth or genital region
12. Rare form of cancer found in AIDS victims
13. Most prevalent STD in the United States today
14. Abbreviation for sexually transmitted disease
15. Received its name in a poem; called the Spanish sickness
16. Protozoan infection affecting the female
17. An STD that is characterized in the male by burning during urination and a pus discharge from the urethra
18. Abbreviation for acquired immune deficiency syndrome
19. Preventive device that may keep one from getting an STD
20. Abbreviation for pelvic inflammatory disease

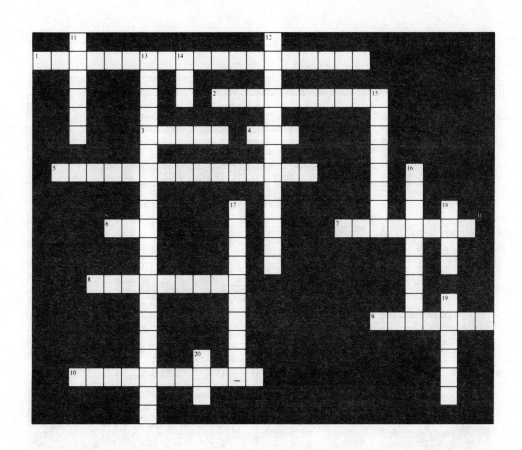

Answer Key to Self-Quizzes

True/False

1. T	6. T	11. T	16. F
2. T	7. F	12. T	17. F
3. F	8. T	13. F	18. T
4. T	9. T	14. T	19. F
5. F	10. F	15. T	20. T

Fill in the Blanks

1. asymptomatic
2. 1
3. chlamydia, gonorrhea
4. rash
5. Flagyl

Crossword Puzzle

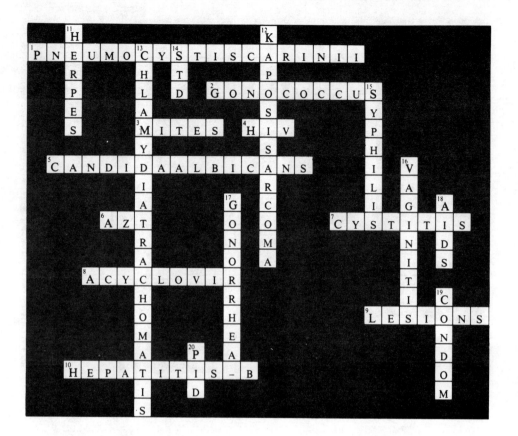

8 Patterns of Sexual Response

According to Masters and Johnson's four-phase model of sexual response, the excitement phase is the beginning of erotic arousal. It may be prompted by thoughts, sights, smells, or the physical contact of foreplay. However, unexpected interruptions, the setting, or numerous other distractions may interfere with the development of sexual excitement. The following is a list of possible distractions. Rate their effect on your level of sexual arousal, using the scale provided.

What Happens to You When . . .

Unexpected Occurrences	Effect on Sexual Excitement		
	Decrease	No Change	Increase
Brightly lighted room			
Expression of love			
Doorbell ringing			
Having an alcoholic drink			
Smell of perfume / after-shave			
Lack of penile erection			
Ears being nibbled			
Having to go to the bathroom			
Soft music playing			
Use of profanity by partner			
Fire in fireplace			
A body massage from partner			
Telephone ringing			
Touching partner's genitals			
Constant unchanging caress			
Showering together			
Lack of vaginal lubrication			
Candlelight dinner			
Rock music playing			
Dog barking			
Unshaved legs / face			
Smell of perspiration on partner			
Being touched on genitals by partner			
Worry about paying the bills			
Use of foam and / or condom			

Reviewing Important Concepts

1. Explain the physiological process of hormones in influencing sexual responsiveness.

2. Sexual response patterns affecting orgasm differ among women and differ for the same woman at different times. List and describe factors that may contribute to this.

3. Describe what happens when a couple attempts simultaneous orgasm.

4. Explain why it is easier for a male than a female to reach orgasm during intercourse.

5. Describe sex differences in regard to the postorgasmic refractory period and multiple orgasms.

Self-Discovery

1. In a survey by Ann Landers, 72 percent of the 100,000 respondents said that they would be willing to forego intercourse if they could be held closely. What can couples do to achieve both orgasm and intimacy with their partners?

2. What experiences were influential in shaping your attitudes toward being sexually receptive toward your partner?

3. Jim and Paula have been in a very committed and loving relationship for over a year. Although it takes Paula a while to reach orgasm, Jim takes great pleasure in knowing that he can orally or manually stimulate Paula to orgasm. Jim, on the other hand, reaches orgasm very quickly. Once he does, his sexual tension has been released, and he doesn't seem to be interested in taking the time that is needed to stimulate Paula to orgasm. What changes would you suggest in Jim and Paula's lovemaking that will take care of their different sexual responses?

4. After a satisfying sexual experience with my partner, I want to . . . , but he or she wants to . . .

5. After orgasm, I feel . . . , and I want my partner to . . .

6. Discuss what is important for you to know about your partner's sexual response.

7. Discuss what you would like your partner to know about your own sexual response.

8. If you are a male, on a sheet of paper describe what you would like every female to know about male sexual response.

9. Psychological factors can contribute greatly to the sexual desire of individuals. Describe those things that you would like from your partner as preliminaries to the sexual encounter to increase your sexual desire.

10. Many people feel uncomfortable about sexual self-stimulation. What are your views on this issue? How can sexual self-pleasuring enhance one's own sexual response?

Self-Quizzes

How well do you know this material? Test yourself by answering the following sample questions.

True/False

_____ 1. Sexual desire arises in a specific part of the brain known as the sexual center.

_____ 2. There are few similarities between two females in regard to the sexual response cycle.

_____ 3. Transudation refers to the moisture that seeps across the vaginal lining and results in lubrication.

_____ 4. The narrowing of the inner third of the vagina is referred to as the orgasmic platform.

_____ 5. The sex flush in the male may occur in either the excitement or plateau phase.

_____ 6. Male orgasm occurs in two stages.

_____ 7. All female orgasms are physiologically the same regardless of the location of the stimulation.

_____ 8. Vasocongestion and muscle tensions reach their peak during the plateau phase.

_____ 9. Both sexes usually experience deep feelings of well-being and relaxation during the refractory phase.

_____ 10. If an individual carefully watches, grades, and compares his or her sexual performance with that of his or her partner, it is called spectatoring.

_____ 11. Both the male and the female use their most erotic sex organ for intercourse.

_____ 12. Male sexuality is more susceptible than female sexuality to psychological influences.

_____ 13. Multiple orgasm in the male is defined as a second ejaculation developing in a short period of time after a first emission.

_____ 14. Simultaneous orgasm is the ultimate sexual experience for a couple.

_____ 15. According to research studies, married couples between the ages of forty and fifty engage in intercourse approximately seven times a month.

_____ 16. Researchers from Duke University found that in the case of older adults, the man was more responsible than the woman for reducing or ending sexual activity.

_____ 17. Individuals who are sexually active in early adulthood are more sexually active in later years.

_____ 18. The availability of a sexual partner is a major obstacle for older men.

_____ 19. Retirement may adversely affect one's sexual functioning.

_____ 20. For some older men, the refractory period may last for twenty-four hours or longer.

Multiple Choice

During the sexual response cycle, both the male and female exhibit physiological changes. Identify which phase is being described in each statement.

Excitement	Plateau	Orgasm	Resolution
A	B	C	D

_____ 1. Strong contractions of the orgasmic platform occur.

_____ 2. Erection of the penis caused by vasocongestion and myotonia occurs.

_____ 3. Coronal ridge swells and turns a deeper reddish purple.

_____ 4. Uterus drops back to normal position.

_____ 5. Clitoris retracts under hood.

_____ 6. Contractions force the seminal fluid through the urethra.

_____ 7. Scrotal sac thins.

_____ 8. Clitoral glans and labia swell because of vasocongestion.

_____ 9. Cowper's gland may release fluid.

_____ 10. Testes increase in size and are fully elevated.

_____ 11. Involuntary muscle contractions occur.

What's Your Sexual Response IQ?

Using the clues that are given, fill in the crossword puzzle. Do not leave a blank space between words.

Across

1. Human process involving emotional, mental, and physical interaction
3. Sexual drive or appetite
5. Retracts under the hood during the plateau phase
9. Spot where some say women ejaculate
10. In males, this brings a feeling of "ejaculatory inevitability"
11. Attained through vaginal stimulation
12. Controls sexual desire in males and females
13. Secretes preejaculatory fluid
15. Marks the beginning of erotic response
17. Increase in blood pressure
19. Hormone secreted by the brain that increases sexual desire
20. Blood flows out through the veins faster than in through the arteries
21. Continuation of events that have occurred during the excitement phase
23. Narrowing of the outer third of the vagina
24. Type of orgasm attained through stimulation of clitoris
25. Two people reaching orgasm at the same time
28. Total response; moves without interruption from phase to phase
29. Spastic contractions of the muscles of the hands and feet (clawlike appearance)
30. When breathing becomes almost twice as fast and deeper

Down

2. Period in which a male cannot achieve another orgasm
4. Sexual gratification
6. Body returns to unaroused state
7. It undergoes contractions during orgasm in the female
8. Engorgement of blood vessels
14. Excessively rapid heart action
16. Reddened, rashlike area of chest, neck, and head
18. One's own unique reaction
22. Speed at which one can be aroused
26. Increased muscle tension
27. Having one orgasm after another during a short period of time

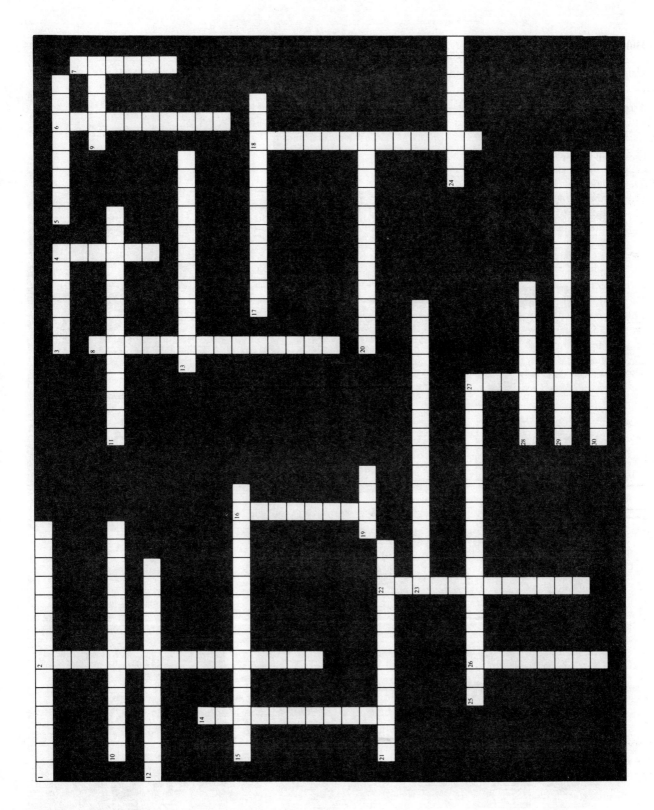

Answer Key to Self-Quizzes

True/False

1. T	6. T	11. F	16. T
2. F	7. T	12. F	17. T
3. T	8. F	13. T	18. F
4. F	9. F	14. F	19. T
5. T	10. T	15. T	20. T

Multiple Choice

1. C	5. B	9. B
2. A	6. C	10. B
3. B	7. D	11. C
4. D	8. A	

Crossword Puzzle

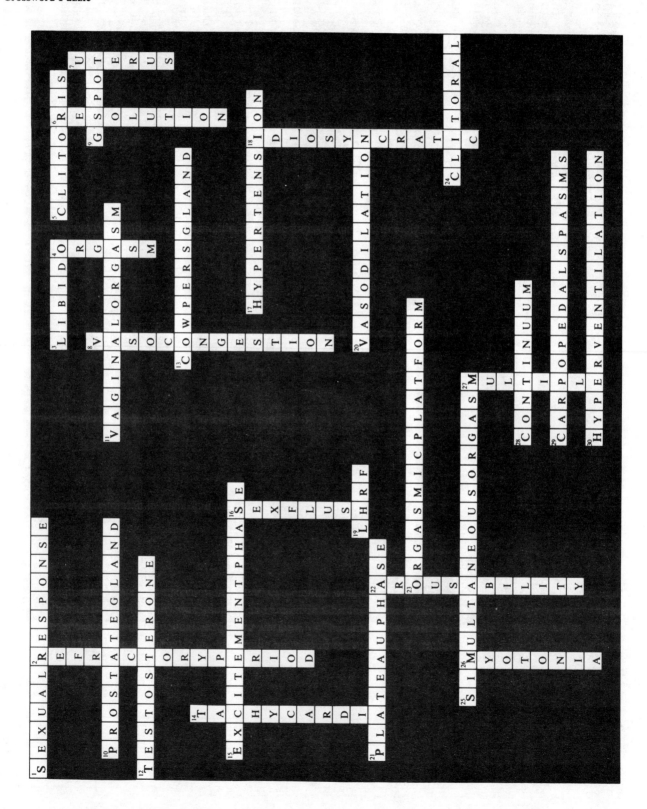

9 Sexual Pleasuring

Arousal is an awakening, a stirring, an unleashing similar to birth in the sense that so many feelings are brought to life. These emotions emerge as a result of many stimuli: a touch, a look, a kiss, a voice, a song, or perhaps even a dream. For some, gentleness and tenderness must be the catalyst; for others a stronger, more passionate approach is desired.

What Is Arousing to You?

Complete the following questionnaire by indicating the degree to which you agree or disagree with each of the statements, using the scale below. There are no correct or incorrect responses to these statements. If you have not experienced the behavior described in the question, then answer whether or not you *think* it would be pleasing to you.

Strongly Agree	Agree	Disagree	Strongly Disagree
1	2	3	4

1. I often have difficulty discussing sex with my partner.   1 2 3 4

2. Sex without love is not enjoyable.   1 2 3 4

3. It is wrong for a couple to engage in any sexual activity that is not enjoyable to both partners.   1 2 3 4

4. I enjoy petting under my partner's clothing.   1 2 3 4

5. Fantasizing increases my sexual excitement.   1 2 3 4

6. Receiving a back rub from my partner is sexually arousing.   1 2 3 4

7. As soon as my partner stands near me, I am attracted to his or her smell.   1 2 3 4

8. I feel comfortable French kissing with someone after just a few dates.   1 2 3 4

9. Manual genital stimulation always results in orgasm for me.   1 2 3 4

10. I would be too embarrassed to go skinny dipping with my partner.   1 2 3 4

11. When my partner nibbles my ears, I want to continue lovemaking until we engage in coitus.   1 2 3 4

12. Taking a bubble bath with my partner is sexually exciting.   1 2 3 4

13. I have no difficulty expressing my sexuality freely and spontaneously.   1 2 3 4

14. Spending a weekend with my partner in a hotel would be the ultimate sexual encounter for me.   1 2 3 4

15. I become sexually aroused when my partner spanks me.   1 2 3 4

16. I enjoy sex the most when my partner describes what he or she is going to do.   1 2 3 4

17. I love it when my partner uses profanity during our lovemaking. 1 2 3 4

18. Self-stimulation is a normal sexual outlet that I enjoy very much. 1 2 3 4

19. There is a significant genital response when my partner stimulates my breasts. 1 2 3 4

20. Oral sex makes me feel totally involved with my partner. 1 2 3 4

21. It is sexually exciting to be held in my partner's arms while dancing. 1 2 3 4

22. I become uncomfortable when I am in a group setting and one or more of the couples engage in intimate behavior. 1 2 3 4

23. I get excited when my partner sucks my fingers or toes. 1 2 3 4

24. I find walking through the woods or on the beach sexually arousing and would enjoy making love outside. 1 2 3 4

25. Watching pornographic movies with my partner is not a sexual turn-on for me. 1 2 3 4

26. Being around someone who is in great physical shape is arousing. 1 2 3 4

27. Oral sex is only pleasing to me if taken all the way to orgasm. 1 2 3 4

28. I enjoy watching my partner touch himself or herself. 1 2 3 4

29. Using a vibrator allows me to discover what is pleasing to me. 1 2 3 4

30. The glow from a fire, candlelight, or soft lighting on my partner's body is more arousing to me than making love in the dark. 1 2 3 4

31. It is very distracting if my partner is too rough or too gentle in stimulating my genitals. 1 2 3 4

32. I feel uncomfortable if I undress in front of my partner. 1 2 3 4

33. Kissing my partner after he or she has smoked a cigarette is a sexual turn-off. 1 2 3 4

34. During self-stimulation, I usually fantasize about someone (not necessarily my partner). 1 2 3 4

35. What my partner is wearing influences my mood. 1 2 3 4

36. Having my partner wake me up in the morning by gently kissing me all over my body is sexually arousing to me. 1 2 3 4

37. Personal hygiene is a prerequisite for my partner and me before an intimate encounter. 1 2 3 4

38. When my partner is pleasuring me and it is not the way I like it, I have difficulty discussing this with him or her. 1 2 3 4

39. Having my partner initiate our lovemaking is sexually stimulating. 1 2 3 4

40. I do not like my partner to wake me up in the middle of the night to make love to me. 1 2 3 4

Reviewing Important Concepts

1. How do the fantasies of males and females differ?

2. Should the genitals be the first or last areas to be caressed? Why?

3. Why has the incidence of cunnilingus and fellatio increased over the past decades? Should you ask your partner to engage in one of these arousal techniques if it is not pleasurable to him or her? Why or why not?

4. Undiagnosed hypertension generally does *not* impair sexual functioning. However, once treatment begins, sexual problems tend to increase. How do you explain this phenomenon?

5. Briefly describe the effects culture and religion have on sexual pleasuring.

Self-Discovery

1. **If you are male** . . .

    a. List in order of importance five parts of the *female* body that you find sexually exciting.

    b. List in order of importance five parts of the *male* body that you *think* a female finds sexually exciting.

    c. List in order of importance *your* five sexiest body parts.

    d. How do your lists in a, b, and c compare?

If you are female . . .

    a. List in order of importance five parts of the *male* body that you find sexually exciting.

    b. List in order of importance five parts of the *female* body that you *think* a male finds sexually exciting.

    c. List in order of importance *your* five sexiest body parts.

    d. How do your lists in a, b, and c compare?

2. If you were asked to fill a brown paper bag with three things that turn you on sexually, what would you put in the bag? Why? (You may *not* include a photograph of your partner.)

3. I become sexually aroused whenever I pleasure my partner by . . .

4. The biggest turn-on for my partner occurs when I . . .

5. I know I can turn off my partner whenever I . . .

6. It would be very difficult or impossible for me to give pleasure to my partner by . . .

7. There is greater variability in female sexual response than male sexual response because . . .

8. Although I would enjoy it very much, I would be embarrassed to ask my partner to . . .

9. I wish my partner would talk to me about . . .

10. The most important sexual organ of the body is the _____ , because . . . .

Self-Quizzes

How well do you know this material? Test yourself by answering the following sample questions.

True/False

____ 1. Touch is the only type of stimulation to which the body can respond reflexively.

____ 2. Sensations that are gratifying are called sensual.

____ 3. Sexual activity that involves self-stimulation is termed autoerotic.

____ 4. Men are much more aroused than women by visual stimulation.

____ 5. Even today some religions view masturbation as a "grave moral disorder."

____ 6. The risk of contracting AIDS through anal intercourse is significantly reduced if you manually dilate the anus before inserting the penis.

____ 7. The coital position favored by most American couples is the woman-on-top position.

____ 8. Although the "missionary" position in coitus has several advantages, it can make it difficult for a woman to move freely.

____ 9. The term *foreplay* is a misnomer because the activities referred to can occur at any stage of sexual activity.

____ 10. Masturbation is experienced by a majority of both sexes, but it is more common among females than males.

____ 11. The preferred frequency of coitus may or may not be the actual frequency.

____ 12. The frequency of intercourse increases the longer a couple live together.

____ 13. The incidence of female masturbation and nocturnal dreams increases after marriage and remains fairly steady even beyond the age of sixty.

____ 14. Potassium nitrate (saltpeter) is an aphrodisiac.

____ 15. The use of marijuana temporarily reduces testosterone levels in the male immediately after smoking.

____ 16. Cocaine is a sex enhancer that prolongs the sexual experience for an hour.

____ 17. Long-term usage of crack leads to an insatiable appetite for sex.

____ 18. "Poppers" are substances that increase sexual desire by creating warm sensations in the genital region.

____ 19. The most common reason women give for faking orgasm is to protect the male's ego.

____ 20. The emotion of anger tends to increase sexual desire.

Fill in the Blanks

1. When the mouth, lips, and tongue stimulate the female's genitals, it is called _____ .

2. _____ , from the Latin word *fellare* meaning "to suck," refers to oral stimulation of the penis.

3. A persistent and painful erection without sexual desire is called _____ and is often induced by the aphrodisiac known as _____ (Spanish fly).

4. Although alcohol and drugs may _____ sexual desire, they may also _____ sexual peformance.

5. A sexual _____ is any daydream having an elaborate script that is sexually exciting.

6. Areas of the body that are particularly sensitive to erotic tactile stimulation are known as _____ .

7. The _____ position in intercourse is useful in overcoming the problem of premature ejaculation.

8. _____ intercourse should not follow _____ intercourse because bacteria from the rectum may cause an infection in the reproductive tract.

9. In low doses, _____ reduce sexual anxiety and sexual inhibitions.

10. In women, the use of _____ may cause a decrease in vaginal lubrication.

Answer Key to Self-Quizzes

True/False

1. T	6. F	11. T	16. F
2. T	7. F	12. F	17. F
3. T	8. T	13. T	18. T
4. F	9. T	14. F	19. T
5. T	10. F	15. T	20. F

Fill in the Blanks

1. cunnilingus
2. Fellatio
3. priapism, cantharidin
4. increase, decrease
5. fantasy
6. erogenous zones
7. lateral
8. vaginal, anal
9. barbiturates or tranquilizers
10. antihistamines

10 Sexuality in Disability and Illness

Sexual health is the integration of the somatic, emotional, mental, and social aspects of sexual being, in ways that are positively enriching and that enhance personality, communication, and love. It is intertwined with our physical health and often has restrictions placed upon it, but it never has to be eliminated from our personhood.

What Would You Do If . . .

Identified below are several real-life situations that may occur to you or a loved one today, tomorrow, or sometime in the future. Complete each of the sentences by placing a rank number (1, 2, 3, 4) in the blank to indicate how you would complete each sentence with the given choices (1 = first choice, 4 = last choice).

1. **If your partner is a male** . . .

   The worst thing that could happen to my sexual partner would be that he
   a. developed diabetes _____
   b. suffered a complete spinal cord injury _____
   c. suffered a heart attack _____
   d. had a prostatectomy _____

   If your partner is a female . . .

   The worst thing that could happen to my sexual partner would be that she
   a. had a mastectomy _____
   b. developed diabetes _____
   c. had a hysterectomy _____
   d. suffered from cerebral palsy _____

2. The worst thing that I could find out about my own sexual health is that I
   a. developed Parkinson's disease _____
   b. suffered a partial spinal cord injury _____
   c. suffered a stroke _____
   d. had cancer _____

3. If my child were blind or deaf, I would
   a. assume all the responsibility for his or her sex education _____
   b. mainstream him or her into a public school so he or she would have normal sexual contacts _____
   c. enroll him or her in a special school that dealt with his or her disability and socialized him or her with other similarly disabled children _____
   d. have our family physician place him or her on birth control immediately _____

4. If my child were mentally handicapped, I would
   a. have our family physician sterilize him or her immediately _____
   b. seek out a school that provided a sex education program that met his or her unique needs and problems _____
   c. assume all the responsibility for his or her sex education _____
   d. enroll him or her in a private institution that separated boys and girls so that sexual contacts would be avoided _____

Medical Complications

Each of the following diseases and disabilities has an impact on one's sexual functioning. The effects are varied and different, ranging from little or no impact to changing one's sexual functioning completely. If you had to suffer from these conditions, which would you be able to accept the easiest and which would be the hardest for you to accept? Rank them accordingly (1 = easiest, 15 = hardest).

a. diabetes _____

b. blindness _____

c. moderate mental handicap _____

d. cerebral palsy _____

e. mastectomy/prostatectomy _____

f. heart attack _____

g. psoriasis _____

h. complete spinal cord injury (quadriplegia) _____

i. partial spinal cord injury (paraplegia) _____

j. ovarian/testicular cancer _____

k. multiple sclerosis _____

l. ileostomy _____

m. Parkinson's disease _____

n. amputation of a leg _____

o. deafness _____

Reviewing Important Concepts

1. Briefly explain why a complete spinal cord injury is less traumatic for a female than a male. Explain how the SCI male may have multiple orgasms.

2. How may sexual experimentation enhance the self-esteem of a person with a disability more than an able-bodied person?

3. If an individual is physically disabled, blind, or deaf at an early age, what is the impact on sexual functioning and communication? How does this differ from an individual who becomes disabled after he or she is married?

4. What inherent problems exist in the "dating game" for a person who is blind? List the mannerisms that such a person exhibits.

5. A vast majority of people who are deaf use sign language to communicate with their family, friends, and lover. How does signing restrict sexual interactions?

6. How can sex education be adapted for people who are mentally handicapped in order to enhance their sexuality in a responsible manner?

7. Why is the decrease of sexual activity among males who have had a heart attack substantially lower than that of females who have had a heart attack of equal severity?

8. What is the primary sexual effect of diabetes on the female? The male? How can these limitations be overcome so the person with diabetes can achieve a satisfying sexual relationship?

9. What is the psychological impact of breast cancer and a hysterectomy on a female? How do women and society view the female breast?

10. What are the risks associated with estrogen replacement therapy?

11. How might an amputation affect a person's sexual self-image?

12. Everyone needs validation as a sexual being. Why is it especially important for a person who has a disability to receive validation?

13. If 96 percent of men who are quadriplegic can gain an erection, then why can only 72 percent have intercourse?

Self-Discovery

1. Should people who are mentally handicapped be given explicit sex education? Why or why not?

2. If your partner were in a car accident and became a paraplegic, how would you handle the situation?

3. If a person who is blind asked to braille your face, would you feel comfortable allowing him or her to do so? Why or why not?

4. Do you feel uncomfortable when you see two individuals signing to each other? Explain.

5. Do you believe people who have mental handicaps should be allowed to have children? Why or why not? If they should not, should they automatically be sterilized, even if it is against their will?

6. If you were engaged and became a quadriplegic, would you break off your engagement? Why or why not?

7. List seven adjectives that *you* associate with people who are disabled. If *you* were disabled, which seven adjectives would you then list?

Self-Quizzes

How well do you know this material? Test yourself by answering the following sample questions.

True/False

_____ 1. In terms of sexual functioning, diabetes is more likely to affect males than females.

_____ 2. Women with spinal cord injuries are capable of producing children.

_____ 3. Odds are if two individuals who are mentally retarded marry and have children, their children will also be mentally retarded.

_____ 4. Breast cancer is usually detected by a physician during a woman's routine gynecological exam.

_____ 5. Prostate cancer is generally found in men under age forty.

_____ 6. Individuals who are disabled are incapable of sexual functioning.

_____ 7. The age at which an individual incurs his or her disability affects that person's socialization.

_____ 8. In a complete spinal cord separation, there is no feeling or movement below the level of separation.

_____ 9. If a male with a spinal cord injury has an erection, then his chances are statistically very good that ejaculation will follow.

_____ 10. The primary factor that research studies have shown to be associated with sexual difficulties following a heart attack is a mental one, fear of suffering another heart attack.

_____ 11. Epilepsy produces a significant neurological reduction in the ability to function sexually.

_____ 12. Following a prostatectomy for cancer, men frequently experience erectile dysfunction.

_____ 13. Testicular cancer is a relatively rare condition in men between the ages of twenty and thirty.

_____ 14. One of the problems associated with being deaf is the inability to "sign" and touch one's partner at the same time.

_____ 15. Full-body function and mobility is impossible for people who are blind or suffer from Parkinson's disease.

_____ 16. People who are mentally retarded are more apt to be exploited sexually than people of normal intelligence.

_____ 17. An oopherectomy is surgical removal of the ovaries.

_____ 18. Cancerous testicles are successfully treated with radiation.

_____ 19. The amputation of a limb may be as psychologically damaging as the loss of a breast or testis.

_____ 20. In relating to a person with a disability, offer help only when requested.

Matching

_____ 1. Dysplasia   A. A skin infection

_____ 2. Breast cancer   B. Loss of sensation in all four limbs

_____ 3. Mastectomy   C. Most commonly occurring form of cancer in women

_____ 4. Pap smear   D. IQ 35–49

_____ 5. Mammography   E. Surgical removal of the breast

_____ 6. Prostate cancer   F. Abnormal cell growth

_____ 7. Psoriasis   G. Second most common form of cancer in men

_____ 8. Colostomy   H. An opening from the intestines

_____ 9. Paraplegia   I. Most reliable means of the early detection of cervical cancer

_____ 10. Moderate mental retardation   J. Loss of sensation in the legs

     K. Low-dose X ray used to screen for breast cancer

     L. IQ 50–70

     M. An opening from the colon

Answer Key to Self-Quizzes

True/False

1. T	6. F	11. F	16. T
2. T	7. T	12. T	17. T
3. F	8. T	13. F	18. F
4. F	9. F	14. T	19. T
5. F	10. T	15. F	20. T

Matching

1. F	6. G
2. C	7. A
3. E	8. M
4. I	9. J
5. K	10. L

11 Sexual Problems and Therapies

Sexual problems can happen to anyone at any time. Difficulties in sexual functioning may be transient or continual. They may be caused by organic factors (illnesses, drugs, or structural abnormalities), psychogenic factors (how we view ourselves and others, as well as how we relate to others), or cultural factors. Individuals may be able to help themselves resolve a sexual difficulty or they may need professional help. Read each case study that follows and answer the questions as if you were the therapist working with each couple.

Case Study 1

Connie and Dan have been married for seven years and have two handsome sons. The couple frequently engaged in sexual intercourse, and both were very satisfied with their level of intimacy. Up until the past eight months, Dan would come home for lunch two or three times a week, and he and Connie would always end up in some type of intimate sexual activity. However, Dan no longer comes home for lunch, and the frequency of their sexual activity has dropped significantly. Connie has become depressed and gained forty pounds. When she tries to initiate their lovemaking, Dan turns away and says he is tired.

a. What sexual dysfunctions may Dan be suffering from?

b. What factors may be contributing to his problems?

c. What can Connie do to help the situation?

d. What specific suggestions would you offer Connie and Dan to improve their sexual relationship?

Case Study 2

Debbie and Bob were engaged for two years before they were married. During their engagement, they enjoyed kissing and light petting, as Debbie was Catholic and said she did not believe in premarital sex. On their honeymoon, Bob noticed that Debbie was unusually tense and her mind seemed to be elsewhere. Feeling that Debbie might be uncomfortable because she was sexually inexperienced, Bob did not push her to have sexual intercourse. It has now been six months since their marriage, and the few times they have tried intercourse, Debbie has said it was not pleasurable. Bob has tried to be gentle and creative in his lovemaking. After the last attempt at intercourse, Debbie pulled away and finally said that her father had abused her.

a. What sexual dysfunction(s) may Debbie be suffering from?

b. What factors may be contributing to her problem(s)?

c. What can Bob do to help their relationship?

d. What specific suggestions would you offer Debbie and Bob to overcome their problem?

Case Study 3

Donna and Jim have lived together for a year and feel that they are sexually compatible. Both enjoy manual and oral stimulation and easily reach orgasm. Jim has had more masturbatory experience than Donna but has confessed that his mother caught and punished him severely. Donna has become disenchanted with their level of sexual intimacy when they engage in sexual intercourse. Although Jim is always satisfied and is able to fall asleep quickly, Donna is not satisfied and becomes angry at Jim's lack of concern.

a. What sexual dysfunction(s) may Jim be suffering from?

b. What factors may be contributing to his problems?

c. What can Donna do to help their relationship?

d. What specific suggestions would you offer Donna and Jim to improve their sexual relationship?

Reviewing Important Concepts

1. List six physical factors associated with erectile dysfunction.

2. How does the fear-of-failure syndrome affect erectile dysfunction?

3. Define ejaculatory incompetence and retarded ejaculation. Identify the physical and psychological causes for these inhibitions.

4. Describe vaginismus. Identify the physical, psychological, and relational problems associated with it.

5. Define spectatoring. How does this contribute to sexual dysfunctions?

6. Trace the phases of sensate focus exercises. Why are they successful in treating some sexual dysfunctions?

7. Identify the organic factors that cause sexual dysfunctioning in men and women.

8. Distinguish between psychogenic factors that are immediate, intrapsychic, and interpersonal.

9. How do cultural expectations and prohibitions contribute to sexual dysfunctioning?

10. How do Masters and Johnson's methods of sexual therapy differ from Kaplan's?

11. Explain the PLISSIT model for therapy.

12. Identify the major training and credentialing agencies for sex therapists in North America.

Self-Discovery

1. How does poor sexual communication contribute to sexual dysfunctions?

2. What are the potential consequences of faking orgasm with your partner? How would you feel if your partner faked orgasm with you?

3. Is the use of surrogate sex partners in therapy simply another form of "white-collar prostitution"?

4. If someone asked you to write the Ten Commandments on "How to Avoid Sexual Dysfunctions," what would you write?

5. Numerous advice columns (Dear Abby, Dear Ann Landers), television programs (Donahue, Dr. Ruth), magazine articles, and popular books offer sexual advice to individuals. In what ways may this information be helpful? Harmful? Would you follow the advice given by one of these sources? Why or why not?

6. A man unable to have an erection is classified as suffering from erectile dysfunction. What should we call it then when he is unable to perform cunnilingus (oral sex)? Is this also a dysfunction? Explain.

7. Would the sex of the therapist influence whether or not the therapy would be successful for you? Why or why not? Would you be more comfortable with a male *and* female therapist? Why or why not?

8. Is it possible that your religious upbringing may contribute to a sexual dysfunction in the future? How?

9. Describe any experiences you had when you were younger that could influence your sexual functioning.

10. How should therapists measure their success rate when dealing with individuals or couples? Which is a better indicator—behavioral changes in the clients or subjective comments by the clients regarding their level of satisfaction? Why?

11. Do you feel that the women's movement and changing gender roles have contributed to an increase in sexual dysfunctions? Why or why not?

12. The term *dysfunction* has replaced the words *impotent* and *frigid*. However, *dysfunction* is a medical term indicating that an organ is unhealthy. Should the phrase *sexual dysfunction* be replaced with *sexual problems?* Why or why not? If it were, do you feel more individuals would seek help for their "problems"?

13. What is the relationship between alcohol and marijuana and sexual dysfunctions? Is either alcohol or marijuana an aphrodisiac? Defend your answer.

14. What, if any, are the advantages of a therapist's treating a homosexual couple rather than a heterosexual couple?

15. **If you are male** . . .
    Have you ever experienced low sexual desire, dyspareunia, erectile dysfunction, and/or premature ejaculation?
       If yes, describe the situation: How did you feel? What do you think caused it? How did your partner react? How did you overcome or treat it?
          Would you ever consider a penile implant? If yes, under what circumstances? If no, why not?

    If you are female . . .
    Have you ever experienced low sexual desire, vaginismus, dyspareunia, general sexual dysfunction, and/or anorgasmia?
       If yes, describe the situation: How did you feel? What do you think caused it? How did your partner react? How did you overcome or treat it?

Self-Quizzes

How well do you know this material? Test yourself by answering the following sample questions.

True/False

____ 1. Sexual difficulties may be related to desire, arousal, and/or orgasm.

____ 2. Treatment for lack of sexual desire has a high success rate.

____ 3. Brailling your partner's body might be a homework assignment given to you by a therapist as part of a sensate focus exercise.

____ 4. A man who has never been able to have sexual intercourse is suffering from secondary erectile dysfunction.

____ 5. Most men who have tried an inflatable penile prosthesis have found it to be too embarrassing and therefore unsatisfactory.

____ 6. Many sexual difficulties reflect conflicts within the relationship.

____ 7. The squeeze technique is used to treat ejaculatory incompetence.

____ 8. Premature ejaculation is usually associated with a psychological problem.

____ 9. Masters and Johnson believe that effective sex therapy requires both a man and woman therapist, so each person has a same-sexed therapist to identify with.

____ 10. Painful intercourse in either the male or female is referred to as anorgasmia.

____ 11. Progressively wider dilators would be used in the treatment of vaginismus.

____ 12. Genital vasocongestion is under the control of the autonomic nervous system.

____ 13. Erectile dysfunction in the male is comparable to orgasmic dysfunction in the female.

____ 14. According to research studies, the number of women who regularly experience orgasm during intercourse is about 60 percent.

____ 15. A woman who may only achieve an orgasm with a partner who has a mustache is suffering from situational orgasmia.

____ 16. Scar tissue from an episiotomy may lead to dyspareunia in the female.

____ 17. Erectile dysfunction is most commonly caused by smoking and alcoholism.

____ 18. Female sexual responses are less sensitive to illness, age, or drugs than the male's.

____ 19. Women who were brought up to believe that sex was "dirty" and only "loose" girls engaged in it, would probably suffer a sexual dysfunction in their adult years.

____ 20. Internal conflicts related to past experiences are called interpersonal conflicts.

Matching

_____ 1. Sexual dysfunctions
_____ 2. Retarded ejaculation
_____ 3. Masters and Johnson
_____ 4. General sexual dysfunction
_____ 5. Dyspareunia
_____ 6. Kaplan
_____ 7. Premature ejaculation
_____ 8. Primary erectile dysfunction
_____ 9. Anorgasmia
_____ 10. Vaginismus

A. Lack of erotic feelings and vaginal lubrication
B. Behavior modification coupled with psychoanalysis
C. The man has never been able to have intercourse
D. Therapy based on behavior modification
E. Disorders that make normal arousal and response difficult
F. Difficulty in reaching orgasm
G. Inability to maintain an erection of sufficient firmness to complete intercourse
H. Delayed vaginal ejaculation
I. Painful intercourse
J. Lack of control over ejaculation during intercourse
K. Involuntary spasms of the vaginal muscles
L. Inhibition of one's sexual appetite

Answer Key to Self-Quizzes

True/False

1. T	6. T	11. T	16. T
2. F	7. F	12. T	17. F
3. T	8. T	13. F	18. T
4. F	9. T	14. F	19. T
5. F	10. F	15. T	20. F

Matching

1. E	6. B
2. H	7. J
3. D	8. C
4. A	9. F
5. I	10. K

12　Biological Sexual Development

Within each person's body are many kinds of cells, but they all carry the same set of genes. Genes act like a blueprint that carries coded instructions for a particular trait or physical characteristic. Have you ever wondered why you have blue eyes and both of your parents have brown eyes? Or why you are 6'4'' and both of your parents are short? The answers to these questions are not obvious, but genetic engineering may soon replace the biologist's explanation of dominant and recessive genes.

Genetic Manipulation

The year is 2025 and the earth has rapidly become overcrowded. In desperation, the World Health Organization has issued a decree stating that each family may only have one child. Genetic engineering has given you and your partner the capability of "selecting" your son or daughter. Tomorrow you are going to the baby lab to select the traits to be associated with your child. You have to decide all of his or her biological characteristics (i.e., gender, health status, eye color, hair color, IQ, race, height, and so forth).

a. Describe your child in as much detail as possible.

b. Which gender would you choose and why?

c. Would your gender choice affect the natural sex ratio that has been relatively stable over time, with slightly more males than females being born?

d. Would the crime rate be affected if many more males than females were born? Why or why not?

e. Would monogamy still exist if one sex greatly outnumbered the other?

f. Would homosexuality increase if people were unable to find partners of the opposite sex?

g. If females outnumbered males, do you think that there would be a female pope? A female president in the United States?

Reviewing Important Concepts

1. Why is there a halving of the number of chromosomes in sperm or ovum production?

2. Who determines the sex of a child? Why?

3. Compare and contrast the development of male and female sex organs. What two hormones are essential to male development? Why? Why aren't female hormones required for the development of the internal female sex organs?

4. Briefly describe the androgen-insensitivity syndrome.

5. Describe the internal and external genitals associated with adrenogenital syndrome.

6. Distinguish between those inappropriately called hermaphrodites and true hermaphrodites.

7. How does the fetal brain become masculinized? What physiological effects does brain differentiation cause during and after puberty?

8. Describe Klinefelter's syndrome. Why is the individual with this syndrome sterile?

Self-Discovery

1. Why aren't parents and children exact copies of one another?

2. Why do you think the male brain is slightly larger and heavier than the female brain?

3. Are the differences in abilities and behaviors between men and women the result of genetics or social conditioning? Explain.

4. In your opinion, what would happen to a male who did *not* have *any* estrogen in his body?

5. If a male received large amounts of estrogen, would this be a useful contraceptive technique? Why or why not?

6. Suppose that in the delivery room you were told that your new baby was a girl, but six weeks later you were informed that tests indicated that your baby was actually a boy. What changes would you make in how you were raising your child?

7. How much of your own maleness or femaleness do you think is determined by chromosomes and hormones and how much is the result of how you were raised and other experiences you have had?

8. Would your view of maleness change if men had menstrual cycles? Why or why not?

9. Men and women share the same hormones, but in varying amounts. Do you feel that variations in a man's emotions or sexual interest may be based on a hormonal cycle or changes in the brain's chemistry? Explain.

10. How is it possible that a single cell is able to develop into a complex thinking organism composed of trillions of cells?

Self-Quizzes

How well do you know this material? Test yourself by answering the following sample questions.

True/False

_____ 1. A person who has the physical characteristics of both sexes is called a hermaphrodite.

_____ 2. Gamete-forming cells are found only in the gonads.

_____ 3. Meiosis is the division of one cell into two.

_____ 4. In most people every body cell contains forty-two autosomes and two sex chromosomes.

_____ 5. The sex chromosomes in a female are two small X chromosomes (XX).

_____ 6. No person has ever been known to survive without having at least one X chromosome.

_____ 7. If at least one Y chromosome is present, the individual will be genetically male.

_____ 8. The critical period for the differentiation of the reproductive structures of the male and female is during the first trimester of pregnancy.

_____ 9. In the male embryo, the Wolffian duct system gives rise to the epididymis, vas deferens, and seminal vesicles.

_____ 10. In the male embryo, the Müllerian duct system gives rise to the penis and scrotum.

_____ 11. The external genitals of both males and females develop from the same embryonic tissues.

_____ 12. A female with only one X chromosome develops "streak" gonads, which function as ovaries.

_____ 13. The secretion of testosterone and Müllerian inhibiting hormone ensures the development of male sex organs.

_____ 14. The Skene's glands are homologous to the Cowper's glands.

_____ 15. Ovarian hormonal activity is required for the development of the female external sex organs.

_____ 16. Females with the andrenogenital syndrome were exposed to excess estrogen while in the uterus.

_____ 17. Females who are classified as androgen-insensitive are sterile.

_____ 18. It is best to let the child with ambiguous sex organs wait until puberty and then choose whether to become male or female.

_____ 19. A karyotype is a chart of a person's chromosomes.

_____ 20. Genes consist of the chemical deoxyribonucleic acid.

Multiple Choice

1. A female with Turner's syndrome
   a. is usually raised as a male.
   b. will be sterile.
   c. tends to be extremely creative.
   d. has an irregular menstrual cycle.

2. A person with Klinefelter's syndrome has which of the following chromosome patterns?
   a. XXY
   b. OY
   c. XYY
   d. XY

3. Which of the following criteria does the Olympic Committee use to determine whether a person may compete in women's events?
    a. female genitalia
    b. less than 5 percent Barr bodies in the cell nuclei
    c. more than 5 percent Barr bodies in the cell nuclei
    d. a female identity

4. Girls who were prenatally exposed to an abnormally high level of androgens and had been raised as girls would probably later show an abnormally
    a. great need for achievement.
    b. great need for taking care of someone else.
    c. high level of feminine interests and behaviors.
    d. high level of masculine interests and behaviors.

5. Which of the following are the sex chromosomes for females and males, respectively?
    a. XO, XY   b. XY, XO
    c. XX, XY   d. XY, XX

Answer Key to Self-Quizzes

True/False   **Multiple Choice**

1. T	6. T	11. T	16. F		1. B
2. T	7. T	12. F	17. T		2. A
3. F	8. T	13. T	18. F		3. C
4. F	9. T	14. T	19. T		4. D
5. F	10. F	15. F	20. T		5. C

13 Gender Identity and Gender Roles

What does it mean to be a man or a woman? Who or what determines how we behave? Our gender identity not only includes the biological aspects of being male or female but also the psychological and sociological influences that affect us daily. No realm of human sexuality is more complex or controversial than our concepts of masculinity and femininity. All societies hold certain expectations for each gender, but whose expectations are right for you?

Gender Roles and Your Personality

Below you will find a list of twenty-five gender-related stereotypes, each portrayed on a nine-point continuum. Circle the number where you think you fall on each stereotype. Try to be honest with yourself. When you are finished, go back and place an *X* where you wish you could be on each characteristic.

1. Very passive   Very active
   1   2   3   4   5   6   7   8   9
2. Very dependent   Very independent
   1   2   3   4   5   6   7   8   9
3. Very emotional   Not emotional
   1   2   3   4   5   6   7   8   9
4. Very subjective   Very objective
   1   2   3   4   5   6   7   8   9
5. Very submissive   Very dominant
   1   2   3   4   5   6   7   8   9
6. Very illogical   Very logical
   1   2   3   4   5   6   7   8   9
7. Very home oriented   Very worldly
   1   2   3   4   5   6   7   8   9
8. Act as a follower   Act as a leader
   1   2   3   4   5   6   7   8   9
9. Do not hide emotions   Hide emotions
   1   2   3   4   5   6   7   8   9
10. Easily influenced by others   Independent thinker
   1   2   3   4   5   6   7   8   9
11. Very nonaggressive   Very aggressive
   1   2   3   4   5   6   7   8   9
12. Very excitable in a minor crisis   Calm in a minor crisis
   1   2   3   4   5   6   7   8   9
13. Not at all competitive   Very competitive
   1   2   3   4   5   6   7   8   9
14. Very indecisive   Very decisive
   1   2   3   4   5   6   7   8   9
15. Cry easily   Never cry
   1   2   3   4   5   6   7   8   9
16. Very insecure   Very self-confident
   1   2   3   4   5   6   7   8   9
17. Very conservative   Very adventurous
   1   2   3   4   5   6   7   8   9
18. Very lackadaisical   Very ambitious
   1   2   3   4   5   6   7   8   9
19. Soft spoken   Use very harsh language
   1   2   3   4   5   6   7   8   9
20. Very talkative   Not at all talkative
   1   2   3   4   5   6   7   8   9

21. Yielding   Stubborn

    1   2   3   4   5   6   7   8   9

22. Very gentle   Very rough

    1   2   3   4   5   6   7   8   9

23. Very neat   Very sloppy

    1   2   3   4   5   6   7   8   9

24. Enjoy art and literature   Dislike art and literature

    1   2   3   4   5   6   7   8   9

25. Easily express tender feelings   Have great difficulty expressing tender feelings

    1   2   3   4   5   6   7   8   9

Scoring

Add up your point total for items 1–18; the score should fall between 18 and 162. A score of less than 64 represents a feminine pole, a score of 64–117 represents an androgynous pole, and a score of more than 117 represents a male pole.

Now add up your point total for items 19–25; the score should fall between 7 and 63. A score of less than 26 represents a female pole, a score of 26–46 represents an androgynous pole, and a score of more than 46 represents a male pole.

a. Overall, how would you describe yourself on items 1–18, feminine, androgynous, or masculine? Now, recalculate your score, using the numbers at which you placed an X. How would you classify yourself this time? If there is a discrepancy in the scores, try to explain the reason for it.

b. How would you describe yourself on items 19–25? Recalculate your score, using the numbers at which you placed an X. Why do you believe that your score changed?

c. Explain why you agree or disagree with the following statement: On questions 1–18, a male pole is more desirable and indicates competency.

d. Explain why you agree or disagree with the following statement: On questions 19–25, a female pole is more desirable and indicates warmth-expressiveness.

e. Complete questions 1–25 above in terms of how *you perceive* your mother's behavior. Did you classify her as feminine, androgynous, or masculine? Repeat the questions one more time, indicating how *you perceive* your father's behavior. Did you classify him as masculine, androgynous, or feminine? How did your parents deviate from traditional gender roles?

f. What messages were you given by your family regarding your appropriate gender role behavior? (Think about the household chores and the toys you were given.) Were these messages more traditional or androgynous?

g. On the basis of the preceding questions, what have you learned about your family and yourself?

Reviewing Important Concepts

1. Indicate whether there really are sex differences in brain differentiation.

2. Identify four socializing agents in the development of gender identity. Which of these has the greatest impact during infancy? Childhood? Adolescence? Adulthood? Why?

3. Putting economic necessity aside, explain why most women prefer to work outside the home.

4. Why should we emphasize the mental similarities between the sexes rather than the differences?

5. How do Doyle's five male gender norms restrict the behavior of a male?

6. Your friend Gary confides in you that he believes he is a female trapped within a male body. Explain the process of sex reassignment.

7. If we were to become totally androgynous in our influences and expectations, how might males and females interact domestically, socially, emotionally, and sexually as a result?

Self-Discovery

1. **If you are male,** what roles are you willing to accept if your wife works outside the home? What roles are you *not* willing to accept? Why?

   If you are female, what roles do you expect your husband to assume if you are to pursue your career? What roles do you *not* expect him to assume? Why?

2. Describe the ideal man. Describe the ideal woman. Which qualities are the same? Different? Why?

3. When I see a man with long hair and an earring, I . . .

4. When I see a woman with very short hair and no make-up or jewelry, I . . .

5. My mother would describe a "real woman" as . . .

6. My mother would describe a "real man" as . . .

7. My father would describe a "real man" as . . .

8. My father would describe a "real woman" as . . .

9. In my opinion, females excel in fine motor coordination and manual dexterity because . . .

10. In my opinion, males excel in gross motor movements because . . .

11. The one thing that is keeping me from becoming androgynous is . . .

12. If I had been born a member of the opposite sex, one thing I would be able to do that I am now unable to do is . . .

13. The biggest disadvantage I would be facing right now if I were a member of the opposite sex is . . .

Self-Quizzes

How well do you know this material? Test yourself by answering the following sample questions.

True/False

_____ 1. Researchers have clearly identified how our gender identity develops.

_____ 2. Through the use of current medical technology, gender identity is readily changed.

_____ 3. Transsexuals see their problem as medical rather than psychological.

_____ 4. In our culture it has traditionally been assumed that women are more emotional and dependent than men.

_____ 5. In our culture men have traditionally been expected to be competitive, assertive, and independent.

_____ 6. The use of violence is viewed as more masculine than using nonviolent means of dealing with conflicts.

_____ 7. More females than males are color-blind.

_____ 8. A beneficial side effect of estrogens is the production of a more favorable ratio of low-density lipoproteins to high-density lipoproteins in the blood, which lowers blood cholesterol levels.

_____ 9. After a stroke, men are more likely than women to suffer language impairments.

_____ 10. Research findings suggest that women respond to stressful situations more quickly than men do.

_____ 11. Recent research has once again confirmed that testosterone is associated with aggression.

_____ 12. Research findings suggest that males have better verbal and language abilities than females.

_____ 13. A greater percentage of body weight is usually fat in males than in females.

_____ 14. Females are better at simple, repetitive tasks; males are better at complex tasks.

_____ 15. Research indicates that the majority of both males and females respond physiologically to erotic material.

_____ 16. Parents and other adults have been shown to treat male and female infants differently because they perceive them differently and have different expectations for them.

_____ 17. A boy who learns how to cook, do laundry, and iron will be criticized by his peers.

_____ 18. Research suggests that the amount of television that children watch may affect their likelihood of exhibiting views on the basis of gender stereotypes.

_____ 19. Since teachers encourage all types of activities and abilities in both boys and girls, teachers make no distinction in the gender roles for boys and girls.

_____ 20. The terms _gender_ and _gender role_ can correctly be used interchangeably.

Fill in the Blanks

1. Any individual or institution that influences a person's values, beliefs, or behaviors is called a(n) _____ .

2. An individual who believes that he or she should have been born a member of the opposite sex is referred to as a(n) _____ .

3. _____ is known with certainty about how we develop gender identity.

4. A general term given to any degree of difficulty with gender identity is _____ .

5. Some people feel that _____ is the single most important shaper of gender roles in the world today.

6. _____ means combining both male and female characteristics.

7. Felice Schwartz, writing in the _Harvard Business Review_, referred to women who chose to remain childless as _____ , and to women who combined family and career as _____ .

8. In _____ , functions such as language ability seem to be fairly evenly divided between the right and left hemispheres of the brain, while in _____ they are more concentrated in the left side.

9. _____ toddlers learn much faster than _____ how to pick up on nonverbal cues from others.

10. On the average, women earn approximately _____ percent of the pay men earn for a similar job.

Answer Key to Self-Quizzes

True/False

1. F	6. T	11. T	16. T
2. F	7. F	12. F	17. T
3. T	8. F	13. F	18. T
4. T	9. T	14. F	19. F
5. T	10. F	15. T	20. F

Fill in the Blanks

1. socializing agent
2. transsexual
3. Little
4. gender dysphoria
5. religion
6. Androgyny
7. career-primary; career and family
8. women; men (females, males)
9. Female; males
10. 60–65

14 Sexual Orientation

Identifying and acknowledging our sexual orientation can and should be exciting and joyful. One of the things that influences the feelings associated with this experience is the existence of a support system, whether it is one person or a network of people. Expressing our thoughts and feelings about ourself as a sexual being can sometimes be difficult unless we can do so with someone who cares about us and loves us *unconditionally* and the lines of communication are truly open. Think about how you would react in the following situation.

Love and War

Luke has always idolized his older brother, Matt, and bragged about him to all his friends at school. Matt had served two tours of duty in Viet Nam, and Luke followed his military career with enthusiasm. He had always hoped to follow in his brother's footsteps and make the military his career as well.

During his first tour of duty, Matt was wounded in combat. While in the hospital, he received his first Purple Heart. After two months of extensive therapy, he returned to Viet Nam for his second tour.

Upon returning to the United States, Matt was given two weeks leave to visit his family and friends. His hometown of Spokane gave him a hero's welcome, complete with a parade and a banquet in his honor. Luke was bursting with pride as he sat with his family and friends at the head table. As he was driving home that night, he couldn't help but think about how he wanted to be just like Matt.

The night before Matt had to report back to duty, he asked Luke if he would help him move into an apartment off base. Luke jumped at the opportunity to spend more time with his brother and visit the base. While they were unpacking Matt's belongings, Luke noticed several pictures of a man he didn't know. It seemed strange to him that there were no pictures of Matt's girlfriend, Sandra, anywhere. When he asked his brother if he and Sandra were still dating, Matt said they were no longer seeing each other. However, he mentioned there was someone "special" in his life that he wanted Luke to meet and invited him for dinner Friday night.

Luke couldn't wait to get to school the next day and tell his friends about his brother's invitation. He wondered what Matt's new girlfriend was like. Maybe Matt was going to announce his engagement and wanted to ask him to be the best man at the wedding. He could see himself now in a tuxedo!

Although dinner was at 7:00, Luke arrived thirty minutes early. After ringing the doorbell, he waited patiently for Matt to come to the door. To his astonishment, the man who opened the door wasn't his brother, but the man in the pictures! What was he doing here? Was this Matt's "special" friend? Phil introduced himself and invited Luke inside.

As the evening progressed, it was apparent that Phil was a very important part of his brother's life. Luke liked Phil right away and found him very easy to talk to. He had never met someone who was so warm and caring, but also strong and athletic. Matt seemed to have a "sparkle" in his eye that he had never seen before. Luke noticed that Matt and Phil almost read each other's mind when one of them wanted or needed something.

Lying in bed that night and trying to sort through his feelings, Luke remembered a statement that his brother had written three months earlier that had made no sense at the time. The statement read, "The United States is the only country that gives you a medal for killing a man, but puts you in jail for loving one." Now Luke understood what Matt was trying to tell him. But how could his own brother be gay? What would happen to Matt if the army found out he was gay? Would his brother go to jail? Would the army even accept Luke if Matt was gay? What would his friends say if they found out? The more Luke thought, the more confused he got.

a. If you were Luke, how would you feel about your brother?

b. Would your brother's homosexuality cause you to question your own sexual orientation?

c. Could you be supportive of your brother's life-style? Why or why not?

Reviewing Important Concepts

1. Why are the results of studies regarding the relationship of hormonal levels to sexual orientation inconclusive?

2. Explain Freud's psychoanalytic theory of homosexuality.

3. By what age is one's sexual orientation usually determined? At what age do people become aware of their orientation? Why is there a difference in these ages?

4. Identify four reasons why people who are primarily homosexual marry.

5. What are the major barriers to coming out and what are some of the expected consequences?

6. In any relationship, does one partner automatically assume a "masculine" (aggressive) role and the other a "feminine" (passive) role? Why or why not?

7. Describe how the civil rights of homosexual people have been limited in this country. Under what laws are homosexual individuals generally prosecuted?

8. Compare and contrast heterosexual and homosexual pleasuring. Are they more similar or different? Why?

9. List five contributing factors to homophobia.

10. Summarize five changes brought about by the gay rights movement since 1960.

Self-Discovery

1. If my best friend confided in me that he or she was gay, I would feel . . .

2. If the person I was dating told me he or she was bisexual, I would feel . . .

3. If my roommate were gay, I would expect him or her to . . .

4. If someone of my own sex made a sexual advance toward me, I would . . .

5. I would feel *comfortable/uncomfortable* in a gay bar because . . .

6. If someone of my own sex asked me to dance, I would . . .

7. If I were invited to a party and knew that most of the guests were homosexual, I would . . .

8. When did you first become aware of your own sexual orientation? Was this a gradual or sudden awareness? Do you still hold some uncertainty about your orientation?

9. Should gay bars and nightclubs be allowed to discriminate against heterosexual patrons? Why or why not?

10. Currently, sodomy is illegal in twenty-four states. Should consenting adults (heterosexuals, bisexuals, and homosexuals) have the right to engage in oral and anal intercourse without the fear of prosecution? Defend your position.

11. Describe the discrimination against homosexual people on your campus. What can heterosexual and homosexual individuals do to foster better understanding between each other?

12. If homosexuality were accepted completely in our culture, would there be a gay life-style? Explain.

Self-Quizzes

How well do you know this material? Test yourself by answering the following sample questions.

True/False

____ 1. Anyone who has had same-sex sexual experience should be considered homosexual.

____ 2. Most heterosexuals have had homosexual fantasies.

____ 3. Research indicates that by the time of adolescence, sexual preference is already determined, even though sexual activity may not have begun.

____ 4. According to Kinsey, most gay men and lesbians are exclusively gay or lesbian in their sexual behaviors.

____ 5. The term *coming out* means that one publicly acknowledges one's gayness.

____ 6. The origins of homosexuality are environmental.

____ 7. An irrational fear of homosexuality is called homophilia.

____ 8. The American Psychiatric Association, in its official *Diagnostic and Statistical Manual of Mental Disorders*, Third edition, Revised (DSM-III), removed homosexuality as a psychiatric disorder.

____ 9. Almost all people who are homosexual are unhappy with their orientation and would become heterosexual if they could.

_____ 10. It is possible to accurately determine a person's sexual orientation by his or her appearance and mannerisms.

_____ 11. The term *lesbian* is associated with the Greek poetess Sappho, who wrote about her love for other women.

_____ 12. Bisexuals are often rejected by both the heterosexual and homosexual communities.

_____ 13. Fathers of male homosexuals tend to be overprotective, dominant, and sexually intimate with their sons.

_____ 14. It is estimated that less than 10 percent of the homosexual population have openly identified themselves as being gay or lesbian.

_____ 15. The chromosomes of homosexual and bisexual people are slightly different from those of heterosexual people.

_____ 16. Lesbians are more likely than gay men to form long-term relationships.

_____ 17. Many states in the United States have legislation prohibiting homosexual acts between consenting adults.

_____ 18. The Stonewall Rebellion marked the beginning of the gay liberation movement.

_____ 19. The U.S. Civil Service Commission has continued its policy of not hiring homosexual people for government jobs.

_____ 20. One of the greatest impediments to enduring homosexual relationships is the lack of social and legal support.

Fill in the Blanks

1. Someone who responds erotically to both males and females and has had sexual interaction with both sexes is called _____ .

2. Most gay and lesbian people come out to _____ first.

3. Apparently, in both heterosexual and homosexual individuals, _____ are more likely than _____ to link sexual activity with emotional intimacy.

4. _____ refers to oral or anal sexual acts or coitus with animals.

5. The term _____ means that people will respond to anything that feels good.

Answer Key to Self-Quizzes

True/False

1. F	6. F	11. T	16. T
2. T	7. F	12. T	17. T
3. T	8. T	13. F	18. T
4. F	9. F	14. T	19. F
5. T	10. F	15. F	20. T

Fill in the Blanks

1. Bisexual
2. Friends
3. Women, men
4. Sodomy
5. *Pansexual* or *omnisexual*

15 Childhood and Adolescent Sexuality

When do we become sexual beings? Up until a century ago, it was thought that our sexual stirrings were dormant until early adulthood. Today, we realize that we are sexual beings from birth. Infants derive sensual pleasure primarily through their mouths, but also through close body contact and their genitals.

Childhood is a crucial and active stage in the development of sexuality marked by curiosity, body exploration, and "special" friendships. Budding romances are seen as early as kindergarten. Adolescence is an explosive time period marked by the physical changes associated with puberty and the psychological conflict of learned values and sexual curiosity.

What Would You Do If . . .

1. You are babysitting for your eight-year-old twin brother and sister and are tucking them into bed. As they kiss you goodnight, they ask if they can ask you some "private" questions. In answering their questions, be sensitive to their age, emotional development, and natural curiosity.

   a. What is sex? Are we old enough to have sex?

   b. When we are in the bathtub, it tingles when we wash ourselves "down there." Why?

   c. Why do Mommy and Daddy kiss so often?

   d. Why does Daddy put his tongue in Mommy's mouth?

   e. Why did Mommy and Daddy get married?

   f. Where do babies come from?

   g. How does the sperm get to the egg?

   h. Where does the baby grow?

   i. How does the baby come out?

   j. Does it hurt to have a baby? Why?

   k. Does it hurt to have sex? Why?

   l. Why was that man in the store holding hands with another man?

   m. Why does Uncle Charlie want to rub his hands all over us? What should we do?

2. You have returned home on summer vacation and discovered that your younger sister is getting ready for her junior prom. She has come to you in confidence with the following questions. In answering her questions, be sensitive to her physical, mental, and emotional maturity and also consider her age, peer pressure, and natural curiosity.

   a. Everyone is planning to go to a beach house unchaperoned after the prom for the weekend. Do you think I should be allowed to go?

   b. Do you think Mom and Dad will let me go?

   c. I'm supposed to take a twelve-pack of beer to the party. Will you buy it for me?

   d. What should I do if my date, Nick, wants me to sleep with him and I don't want to? How can I not be embarrassed? Will he still love me?

   e. If I really love Nick, is this the right time to have sex?

   f. Will I find out if I am in love with Nick if I have sex with him?

g. What should I do to keep from getting pregnant? What form of birth control would you recommend?

h. Will I get pregnant if he "pulls out" before he ejaculates?

i. Can I get AIDS?

j. How can I prevent getting a disease?

Reviewing Important Concepts

1. Give an example of a negative childhood sexual experience that is still vivid in your mind. What message did your parents verbally or nonverbally give you regarding this experience? How would you handle this differently with your own child?

2. It is harmless for children of the same sex or opposite sex to examine each other's genitals while playing "doctor." Why do you agree or disagree?

3. If your seven-year-old child saw you and your partner engaging in sexual intercourse, what would you say to the child? Would you be embarrassed? Why or why not?

4. What effect does the media have on the self-concept of an adolescent?

5. Why might first intercourse be perceived as one of life's peak experiences or a major disappointment?

6. Do you agree that gender role behavior and sexual orientation are separate personality elements? Explain. Is an adolescent homosexual encounter predictive of a homosexual life-style?

7. Identify and explain three causes of adolescent pregnancy. What do you feel is the most effective way to reduce the incidence of adolescent pregnancy?

8. Parents tend to wait to tell a child about "the facts of life" until the child is "old enough" to understand, only to find out that doing so is either too embarrassing or the child already knows. What age is the most appropriate for developing attitudes and teaching a child about sexuality? How would you begin?

Self-Discovery

1. Because self-exploration seems to be an important aspect of sexual development, should children actually be encouraged to explore their own genitals? Why or why not?

2. If you were a parent and discovered that your own teenager was sexually active, how would you feel? Would your response be different for your son than for your daughter?

3. Do you feel offering contraceptives in a high school setting is appropriate? Why or why not? Design some guidelines for such a program.

4. Whenever I saw my parents fighting I felt . . . , because . . .

5. The funniest thing that I believed about sex as a child was . . .

6. The earliest childhood sexual experience I can remember with a person of the same sex is . . .

7. The earliest childhood sexual experience I can remember with a person of the opposite sex is . . .

8. An adolescent sexual experience I can remember with a person of the same sex is . . .

9. An adolescent sexual experience I can remember with a person of the opposite sex is . . .

10. I always felt uncomfortable when I saw my parents . . .

11. **If you are female** . . .

    If I got pregnant as a teenager, I would . . .

    If you are male . . .

    If I were a teenager and fathered a child, I would . . .

Self-Quizzes

How well do you know this material? Test yourself by answering the following sample questions.

True/False

_____ 1. Many parents deal with their children's sexuality the same way that their parents dealt with their sexuality.

_____ 2. Infants rarely experience a diffused sort of pleasure from genital stimulation.

_____ 3. Childhood masturbation should not be a source of alarm for parents.

_____ 4. According to child development authorities, the most significant role models in a child's life are his or her parents.

_____ 5. At birth, male testes grow rapidly until puberty.

_____ 6. Gynecomastia usually disappears without treatment during puberty.

_____ 7. Male puberty begins at an earlier age than female puberty.

_____ 8. Breast size is related to sexual adequacy.

_____ 9. Upon the onset of menstruation, a female may experience irregular periods for approximately one year.

_____ 10. Adolescent marriages are associated with lower lifetime earnings because of a lack of formal education.

_____ 11. Adolescent sexual fantasies and activity reflect an individual's true sexual orientation.

_____ 12. Most Americans favor school- and community-based programs to reduce adolescent pregnancy.

_____ 13. According to Stark, the most common reason for adolescent females to have intercourse is sexual gratification.

_____ 14. In 1989, the U.S. Supreme Court delegated individual states more power to regulate abortion.

_____ 15. Sex produces instant adulthood.

_____ 16. Effective sex education includes training in decision-making skills.

_____ 17. Sex education contributes to total self-esteem and more rewarding sexual relationships.

_____ 18. Childhood sex play is abnormal, and children who engage in such activities should be taken to a psychologist.

_____ 19. Parents who are comfortable with their own sexuality are more likely to perceive their children's sexuality in a positive manner.

_____ 20. Because of the deep emotions attached to petting, it always leads to vaginal intercourse.

Fill in the Blanks

1. The period from the onset of puberty to adulthood can be defined as _____ .

2. Books, photographs, or films intended to cause sexual excitement are deemed _____ .

3. The word *psychosexual* pertains to the _____ aspects of sexuality.

4. _____ usually takes two to four years and is indicated by great physical and psychological changes.

5. The term used to describe females who have no ovulatory cycle is _____ .

Multiple Choice

1. Many infants develop methods of masturbation for which of the following reasons?
   a. as a source of pain
   b. as a source of pleasure
   c. to relieve loneliness
   d. to gain acceptance

2. According to Erikson, the greatest developmental task in adolescence is the development of:
   a. intimacy
   b. productivity
   c. industry
   d. identity

3. During puberty, males experience all of the following EXCEPT:
   a. testes grow rapidly
   b. penis grows in length and diameter
   c. body weight and height increase
   d. hormone levels decrease

4. The incidence of adolescent marriage has:
   a. sharply declined
   b. sharply risen
   c. remained constant
   d. slightly risen

5. Causes of adolescent pregnancy include all of the following *except*
   a. low self-esteem.
   b. limited dating experiences.
   c. positive role models.
   d. limited awareness of life's options.

Answer Key to Self-Quizzes

True/False

1. T	6. T	11. F	16. T
2. F	7. F	12. T	17. T
3. T	8. F	13. F	18. F
4. T	9. T	14. T	19. T
5. F	10. T	15. F	20. F

Fill in the Blanks

1. adolescence
2. pornographic
3. emotional
4. Puberty
5. *anovulatory*

Multiple Choice

1. B
2. D
3. D
4. A
5. C

16 Adult Sexuality

For many, the transition from adolescence to adulthood is long and slow, seen clearly only in hindsight. The greatest challenge of adulthood is the formation of intimate relationships, both sexual and nonsexual. Although intimate relationships can enrich your life and enhance your self-concept, they can also leave you feeling exposed and vulnerable. The following poem invites you to think about *your* needs now that you have reached adulthood.

What Do You Need?

I need the laughter we share when we are being silly.
I need the love we feel when we're being serious.
I need the arguments we have to get rid of angry feelings.
I need the look in your eyes, that melts my heart.
I need you to be my friend, when I'm feeling lonely.
I need the craziness, happiness, and even the loneliness of being in love with you.
But most of all, I need you to love me.

Author unknown

1. Which line(s) of this poem is (are) the most meaningful to you? Why?

2. Which need mentioned in the poem do you have now that you did not have during adolescence? Why?

3. Which of the needs noted in the poem would you have a difficult time expressing to the significant other person in your life? Why?

4. Which line(s) of the poem is (are) the most meaningful to your partner? Why?

Reviewing Important Concepts

1. Compare and contrast a single life-style with cohabitation.

2. Briefly explain five criteria that may indicate whether or not an individual is ready for marriage.

3. Identify the individual who is likely to be in an abusive relationship.

4. Explain the personal, social, economic, and sexual adjustments that occur with marriage.

5. Briefly explain five factors that contribute to sexual infidelity in marriage.

6. Currently, one out of two marriages ends in divorce in the United States. What factors in our society have caused the steady increase in the divorce rate?

7. Describe the physiological changes of the climacteric associated with both sexes.

8. For some people, approaching the midlife years promotes anxiety about losing their youth. What are some of the positive aspects of one's sexual activity during midlife?

9. Describe how the sexual response cycle differs in older men and women in comparison to their younger counterparts.

10. Why are midlife remarriages often more successful than earlier marriages?

11. Describe the unique problems of middle-aged widowhood.

12. How do nursing home practices negatively affect the sexual expression of their elderly residents?

Self-Discovery

1. If someone asked you for some tips on how to remain sexually fit, what suggestions would you make?

2. How would you deal with the discovery that your partner is having an affair?

3. No one person in a partnership is responsible for infidelity in the relationship. Instead of its being destructive, how might this experience bring a relationship back into a strong union?

4. Couples divorce each other, not their children. How can children maintain relationships with both parents instead of feeling alienated by one or both?

5. If your parents were to divorce, how do you think you would accept their dating other people?

6. What do you want for yourself in your career and in personal relationships at age forty? At age fifty? At age sixty? At age seventy?

7. Midlife crisis is not brought about by one specific incident and is not predominantly a male syndrome. What can you do throughout your life in an attempt to approach the midlife years with a greater sense of fulfillment and satisfaction rather than of questioning and doubting?

8. Describe yourself as a "sexy senior citizen."

9. How does the media's image of sexiness affect how older adults perceive themselves as sexual beings?

10. You have just been hired as an administrator at a nursing facility. What new policies would you initiate in order to enhance the residents' sexual behavior?

11. If my partner asked me to move in with him or her, I . . .

12. I am *in favor of/against* living together before marriage because . . .

13. If my partner died unexpectedly at age forty-five and I had children, I would . . .

14. If I had been married three years and was unhappy with my marriage, I would . . .

15. If I had been married ten years, had two small children, and was unhappy with my marriage, I would . . .

16. After forty years of marriage, my grandparents have just announced that they are going to be divorced. I am . . .

17. When I see an older couple holding hands or kissing, I feel . . .

18. When I think about getting old, I feel . . .

19. If my partner physically abused me, I would . . .

20. The most stressful aspect of being a new parent would be . . .

Self-Quizzes

How well do you know this material? Test yourself by answering the following sample questions.

True/False

____ 1. The opposite of intimacy is emotional isolation.

____ 2. In a continuing relationship, the level of intimacy remains the same from day to day and year to year.

____ 3. Intimate relationships with others is accomplished only after our self-identity is established.

____ 4. Self-actualization places an increased emphasis on interpersonal relationships.

____ 5. As a partnership develops, it is necessary to keep the lines of communication open.

____ 6. Shared intimacy is an important phase of a fulfilled life-style.

____ 7. Women adjust to a second marriage better than men do.

____ 8. People who choose a single life-style are generally happier and live longer than those who marry.

____ 9. Cohabitation usually refers to unmarried individuals living together in a sexual relationship.

____ 10. The average age of first marriage has decreased in recent years.

____ 11. Commitment and companionship are two criteria for a successful marriage.

____ 12. Even today, women feel the need to marry for financial security.

____ 13. Couples living together do not have the same tax breaks that married couples have.

____ 14. Married women who have a full-time career feel less stress than single women because their spouses share household responsibilities with them equally.

____ 15. Most authorities view infidelity as one of the results of marital deterioration.

____ 16. Menopause usually occurs between the ages of fifty and sixty.

____ 17. The better one's health in the early years, the greater one's enjoyment in the midyears.

____ 18. The midlife years are critical in marital relationships.

____ 19. As a person grows older in years, his or her sex drive diminishes.

____ 20. Women are less orgasmic during middle age than when they were younger.

Fill in the Blanks

1. About _____ percent of Americans will marry at least once.

2. The _____ of aging is not well known.

3. Intimate relationships are a necessary part of _____ .

4. Divorce alternatives include _____ and _____ .

5. After menopause, the ovarian production of the hormones _____ and _____ decreases.

Multiple Choice

1. Singles now make up approximately what percentage of the population?
   - a. 60 percent
   - b. 50 percent
   - c. 20 percent
   - d. 40 percent

2. Traits that produce happy marriages include a sense of humor, concern for the needs of others, and which of the following?
   - a. the ability to adjust
   - b. selfishness
   - c. jealousy
   - d. partnership

3. A lack of communication is indicative of which of the following?
   - a. weakness in one of the partners
   - b. a relationship that lacks emotional intimacy
   - c. constant arguments
   - d. loneliness

4. Physical abuse can be attributed to which of the following?
   - a. a cycle of violence
   - b. stress
   - c. drug abuse
   - d. all of the above

5. Successful parenthood requires which of the following?
   - a. lots of money
   - b. practicality
   - c. emotional stability
   - d. high status

Answer Key to Self-Quizzes

True/False

1. T	6. T	11. T	16. F
2. F	7. F	12. F	17. T
3. T	8. F	13. T	18. T
4. F	9. T	14. F	19. F
5. T	10. F	15. T	20. F

Fill in the Blanks

1. 70
2. biology
3. self-actualization
4. counseling, temporary separation
5. estrogen, progesterone

Multiple Choice

1. D
2. A
3. B
4. D
5. C

17 Birth Control and Abortion

Although sexual intercourse has reproduction as its goal some of the time, it is often used solely as an expression of intimacy. Civilized humans have practiced conception control since the beginning of recorded time for this very reason. Margaret Sanger, a pioneer in the birth control movement in the United States, once said, "No woman can call herself free who does not own and control her body. No woman can call herself free until she can choose consciously whether she will not be a mother" (*Parade,* Dec. 1, 1963). Do you agree or disagree?

Conception Control

Complete the following questionnaire by indicating the degree to which you agree or disagree with each of the statements, using the scale below. There are no correct or incorrect responses to these statements.

Strongly Agree	Agree	Disagree	Strongly Disagree
1	2	3	4

1. Health clinics should be established in junior and senior high schools to provide birth control.   1 2 3 4

2. People generally have a good idea how easy it is to get pregnant.   1 2 3 4

3. The reason there is no male contraceptive available today is because most of the researchers are men who only want to work on methods for use by women.   1 2 3 4

4. Legal abortions are safer than full-term pregnancies.   1 2 3 4

5. Improved birth control methods have lead to an increase in cohabitation among couples.   1 2 3 4

6. Availability and cost are the two most important factors in choosing a method of birth control.   1 2 3 4

7. Religion plays a smaller role in a couple's decision to use birth control today than it did previously.   1 2 3 4

8. The government should fund abortions through Medicaid.   1 2 3 4

9. The man should insert the diaphragm as part of foreplay.   1 2 3 4

10. Birth control pills are safer today than they were twenty years ago.   1 2 3 4

11. It is unethical for the United States to ship birth control products that have been banned by the FDA to Third World countries.   1 2 3 4

12. The cycle of poverty in the United States is being perpetuated by the soaring teenage pregnancy rate.   1 2 3 4

13. The female should unroll the condom over the erect penis during foreplay.   1 2 3 4

14. Males should share equally in the cost of the chosen birth control method.   1 2 3 4

15. The longer a person uses a particular birth control method, the less effective it becomes.   1 2 3 4

16. If a couple decides on sterilization as their birth control technique, the man should undergo a vasectomy.   1 2 3 4

17. Considering the birth control methods available to most American men and women today, the pill is the most effective and has the fewest side effects for most women.   1 2 3 4

18. The contraceptive sponge of the 1980s is as revolutionary for the female as the condom was for the male.   1 2 3 4

19. Spermicides are too messy to use.   1 2 3 4

20. Genetic disorders could eventually be eliminated through the use of birth control.   1 2 3 4

21. An antipregnancy vaccine would be welcomed by women.   1 2 3 4

22. The IUD is an abortion technique.   1 2 3 4

23. College couples do not use contraceptives because they do not want to appear prepared for the possibility of sexual intercourse.   1 2 3 4

24. Natural family planning is only effective if the couple have good communication skills.   1 2 3 4

25. Douching immediately after sexual intercourse reduces the chances of an unwanted pregnancy.   1 2 3 4

What's Your Decision?

A woman may decide to have an abortion for many different reasons. Indicate which of the following reasons you could be the most supportive of by placing its number in the appropriate place on the continuum. The farther you place your number to the left, the more supportive you are of the decision to have an abortion.

For -- Against

1. Incest — Alcoholic and abusive father gets thirteen-year-old daughter pregnant.
2. Mental instability — Woman is grieving over her baby who died of sudden infant death syndrome three weeks ago.
3. Age — Fifty-year-old woman is afraid her baby will have a birth defect.
4. Economics — Unemployed and unskilled woman with three other children becomes pregnant.
5. Rape — Twenty-two-year-old married black female is raped by white male.
6. Health — Woman has had X rays and extensive medication through her second month of pregnancy.
7. Life-style — Married woman wants to complete medical school.
8. Marital difficulty — Woman has filed for legal separation from her husband.

Reviewing Important Concepts

1. Briefly summarize seven reasons for birth control.

2. What are seven criteria for selecting an appropriate method of birth control? Which two are the most important and why?

3. Compare and contrast the theoretical effectiveness and the actual use effectiveness of a birth control technique.

4. Describe the typical U.S.-made rubber condom. How does it differ from the skin condom? If a condom bursts during its use, what can be done to help avoid conception?

5. Why is there more hope for gossypol as an acceptable male birth control pill than for other birth control drugs that have been previously researched?

6. Why are there more birth control devices for women than for men?

7. Describe the female who should *not* take the pill and indicate why she is at a greater-than-average risk for developing serious medical complications.

8. How do the minipill, morning-after pill, and injectable hormones differ in action and content from the combination pill?

9. What were the side effects of diethylstilbestrol (DES), a drug taken from the 1940s through the 1960s to prevent miscarriage?

10. Why have nearly all IUDs been removed from the U.S. market?

11. What characteristics of the contraceptive sponge distinguish it from the diaphragm and cervical cap? Which of these devices is the most effective and why?

12. When does ovulation occur? How can a woman determine her "fertile" period on the basis of the rhythm method?

13. How does a woman's body temperature change when she ovulates? What is basal body temperature?

14. Describe the changes that occur in vaginal mucus secretions when a woman ovulates.

15. Summarize the sympto-thermal method of birth control. Why would it be more reliable than the other methods of natural family planning?

16. After a vasectomy, how long will a man remain fertile? Why? How are the sex drive and the amount of semen affected?

17. Describe the procedures used in vacuum aspiration, dilation and curettage, dilation and evacuation, and induction abortions. Which procedure is the safest and why?

18. How does a saline injection differ from a prostaglandin injection?

19. Summarize the physical and psychological complications of an abortion on both the mother and father.

20. Explain the legal status of abortion in the United States.

Self-Discovery

1. If your best friend were sexually active on a regular basis, would you try to convince him or her to use birth control? Why or why not?

2. Would the fact that a birth control method was or was not reversible be of significance to you? Why?

3. If you and your partner abstained from all physical intimacy for three months, would it dull or intensify your sexual yearning for each other? Why?

4. If you and your partner were considering sterilization, how would you decide who would be sterilized?

5. A close friend of yours has just confided to you that she is pregnant. She is nineteen years old, a college freshman, and unemployed. What advice would you give her and why?

6. In your opinion, do males view birth control differently than females? If so, how? Why?

7. Do teenagers choose a birth control method differently than single or married women? Why?

8. Should young couples consider sterilization as a means of birth control? What might be the future consequences?

9. Is abortion a birth control method? Why or why not?

10. If your sixteen-year-old daughter asked you to recommend a birth control method, what advice would you give her?

11. If an effective birth control pill for men were developed, would most men be willing to use it? How would society have to change the socialization of men for them to be receptive to assuming the responsibility for conception control?

12. In a country where there are not enough resources to handle the population, should the government be allowed to mandate strict family planning programs?

13. Should the United States government fund all abortions? Explain.

If You Are Sexually Active . . .

1. Are you using birth control regularly? Why or why not?

2. If you are using birth control, which method are you using and why? How did you and your partner decide on this method? How do you share responsibility for it?

3. When I forget to use our birth control technique, I feel . . . and I wish we would only engage in . . .

4. I wish my partner would assume more responsibility for conception control by . . .

5. The thought of becoming pregnant right now is . . .

6. If I became pregnant, the first person I would tell is . . . because . . .

7. If my mother were to become pregnant right now, I would feel . . .

8. I am not sure I (or my partner) could undergo an abortion because . . .

9. The father of an unborn child *should/should not* have the right to deny an abortion because . . .

10. If a good friend asked me to go with her to have an abortion, I would . . .

Self-Quizzes

How well do you know this material? Test yourself by answering the following sample questions.

True/False

_____ 1. Oral contraceptives are the most effective reversible means of preventing pregnancy.

_____ 2. Progestaserts are plastic T-shaped devices that have been saturated with estrogen.

_____ 3. Sterilization has become the most commonly used form of fertility control among married couples in the United States.

_____ 4. The most effective barrier method of birth control is the use of spermicidal foam or cream.

_____ 5. The cervical cap fits snugly over the cervix and may be left in place for twenty-four hours.

_____ 6. IUDs are effective because they interfere with the level of estrogen and progesterone that is released.

_____ 7. Spermicidal foams, jellies, and creams must be applied no more than one hour before intercourse.

_____ 8. A diaphragm must be carefully fitted to the individual woman by a doctor or nurse-practitioner.

_____ 9. When using condoms, it is important never to use vaseline or petroleum jellies with them.

_____ 10. Cervical mucus secretions are usually cloudy during ovulation.

_____ 11. Depo-Provera has been approved by the FDA for use as a contraceptive in the United States.

_____ 12. Unlike the diaphragm, the contraceptive sponge contains a spermicide.

_____ 13. Douching increases the chances of vaginal infections but decreases the chances of pregnancy and sexually transmitted diseases.

___ 14. The female hormone progesterone causes a noticeable rise in temperature the day after ovulation.

___ 15. The most common method of female sterilization is tubal ligation.

___ 16. During the first three months of pregnancy, the decision to abort an embryo lies with the woman and her physician.

___ 17. According to *Webster* v. *Reproductive Health Services,* physicians were required to test for the viability of a fetus at twenty weeks.

___ 18. Dilation and Curettage (D and C) accounts for almost 94 percent of all abortions performed in the United States.

___ 19. The safest instillation solution is saline.

___ 20. RU-486 is the newest drug approved by the FDA that interrupts pregnancy in its early stages.

How Much Do You Know?

Using the clues that are given, fill in the crossword puzzle. Do not leave a blank space between words.

Down
1. Lowest body temperature of a person who is awake
2. Sperm killing
3. Noncoital sex
4. Injectable progestin
5. Fits inside uterus to prevent pregnancy
6. Removal or expulsion of a growing embryo
7. Progestin-only pill
8. Prophylactic
9. Technique by which contents of the uterus are sucked out
10. Male birth control pill
11. Device subject to a worldwide recall
12. Those who contend that a growing embryo is human
13. Combines the BBT method with the mucus method
14. Small, thimble-shaped device that fits over the cervix
15. Male sterilization
16. A medicated IUD
17. Shallow, round dome placed to cover the cervix

Across
18. Surgical incision into the uterus to remove fetal/placental contents
19. The most effective method of conception control aside from total abstinence
20. Synonym for a miscarriage
21. What should precede any abortion decision
22. Fertility awareness
23. Hypothetical, abstract
24. Insertion of lighted telescope through dome of the vagina
25. Abbreviation for a disease caused by complications of an IUD
26. Often known as menstrual regulation
27. Effectiveness when used under everyday conditions
28. Diethylstilbestrol
29. Type of IUD wrapped in copper
30. No sexual intercourse
31. Removal of uterus
32. Small, pillow-shaped polyurethane pad
33. Pill that contains synthetic estrogen and progestin
34. Insertion of lighted telescope through abdominal wall
35. Removal of both testes
36. Withdrawal of penis from vagina prior to ejaculation

Answer Key to Self-Quizzes

True/False

1. T	6. F	11. F	16. T
2. F	7. T	12. T	17. T
3. T	8. T	13. F	18. F
4. F	9. T	14. T	19. F
5. T	10. F	15. T	20. F

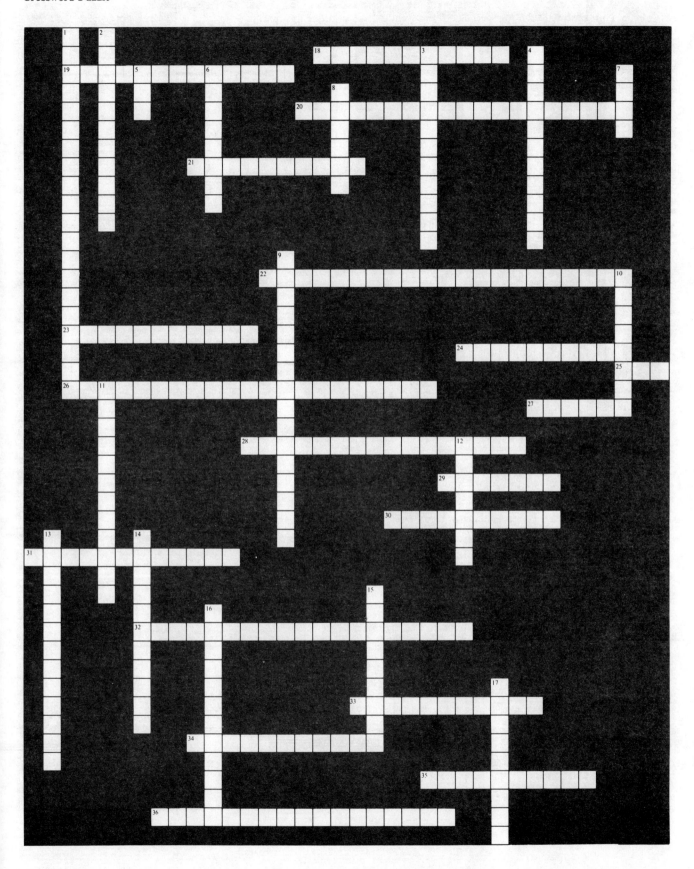

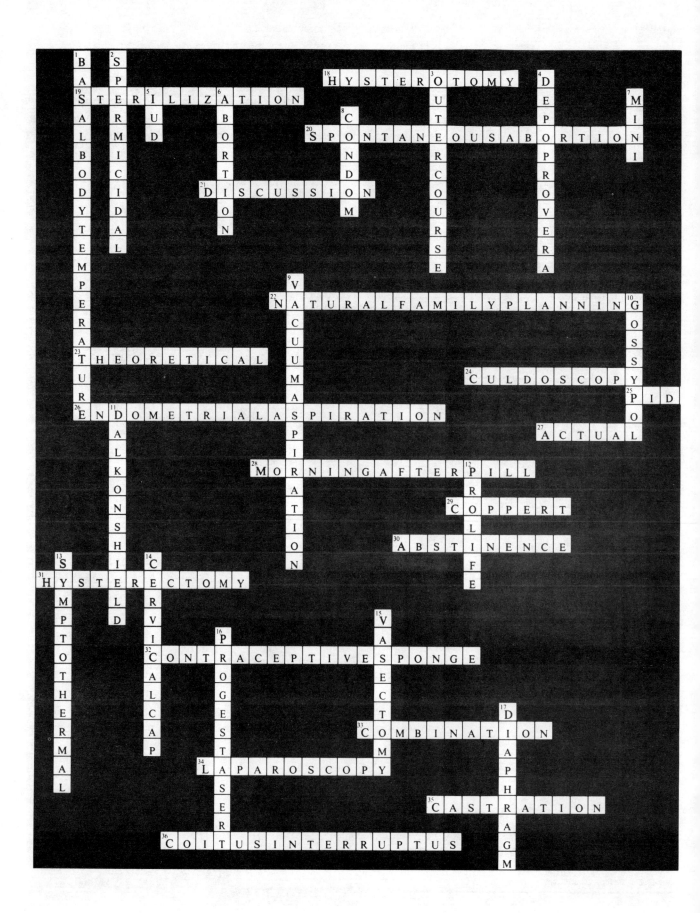

18   Conception, Pregnancy, and Birth

Contraceptive technology has revolutionized today's family. Couples can become parents by choice rather than chance, or they may remain childless. Although two-thirds of all married couples say they want children, the childless alternative has become more socially accepted since World War II. Kahlil Gibran, a noted philosopher and poet, wrote the following about children in his book *The Prophet:*

On Children

Your children are not your children.
They are the sons and daughters of Life's longing for itself.
They come through you but not from you,
And though they are with you yet they belong not to you.
You may give them your love but not your thoughts,
For they have their own thoughts.
You may house their bodies, but not their souls,
For their souls dwell in the house of tomorrow, which you cannot visit, not even in your dreams.
You may strive to be like them, but seek not to make them like you.
For life goes not backward nor tarries with yesterday.
You are the bows from which your children as living arrows are sent forth.
The archer sees the mark upon the path of the infinite, and He bends you with his might that His arrows may go swift and far.
Let your bending in the Archer's hand be for gladness;
For even as He loves the arrow that flies, so He loves also the bow that is stable.

1. Do you agree with Gibran's description of children? Why or why not?

2. Which lines(s) of this poem is (are) the most meaningful to you? Why?

3. Which part of this poem would your mother agree with the most and why? Your father and why?

Parenting by Choice

1. There are good and bad, personal and religious, logical and illogical, thoughtful and selfish reasons for having a child. Listed below are some of the reasons that couples generally identify. Put an *X* by the five most important reasons for *you* to have a baby. Put two stars by the five reasons that you would *never* use as the basis for determining to have a child.

   a. To strengthen the relationship I have with my partner
   b. To please my family and friends
   c. For personal identity
   d. Because I can financially afford a child
   e. Because I already have a son and I want a daughter, or vice versa
   f. Out of fear of being alone in my old age
   g. To be loved
   h. To relive my own childhood
   i. Because my closest friends have recently become parents
   j. To be needed by someone
   k. To be proud of my child's accomplishments
   l. Because of a religious influence
   m. For personal fulfillment
   n. To carry on the family name
   o. Because *my partner* wants to have a child
   p. To escape from the outside working world and stay at home
   q. To prove that I can be a better mother or father than my parents were
   r. Because I am going to be available, not busy
   s. Because I want the challenge of raising a healthy child
   t. To save a deteriorating relationship with my partner
   u. Because *I* want to have a child

2. Do any of your answers to question 1 surprise you? If so, which ones?

3. On the basis of your answers to question 1, do you feel you are ready to have children right now? Why or why not?

4. Would your answers be any different if you projected yourself five years into the future? How? Why?

Dear Vicki

You have just been hired by a large newspaper to respond to individuals who have personal problems. Read each letter and decide what advice you would give each person.

Dear Vicki,

Alex and I have been married five years and we cannot have children. We are both in our early thirties, and all of our friends have started a family. We are beginning to be included less and less with our friends who have children, and we feel left out. Should we consider adoption?

signed,
Liz

Dear Vicki,

I am a twenty-nine-year-old male who desperately wants to have children, but I am sterile. My best friend looks a lot like me, is healthy, athletic, and very intelligent. I would like to have him donate his sperm to impregnate my wife, Sandra. How can I convince Sandra that it would not be "his" baby but "our" baby?

signed,
Guy

Dear Vicki,

Patti and I have been happily together for eight years. We are professionally employed and have strong family feelings. The only thing lacking in our relationship is a child. A good male friend has volunteered his sperm to impregnate one of us. How do we decide which one of us should carry the baby?

signed,
Kim

Dear Vicki,

I am a healthy forty-five-year-old who is pregnant. My husband Larry is sixty-four, and we already have three grown children. I have always loved children, and I am excited about starting another family now that we are financially secure and can spend more time with our baby. Larry does not want the baby, as he says he will be eighty-two when the child graduates from high school. What should I do?

signed,
Rosemary

Dear Vicki,

Janice and I have been going steady for two years, and we just found out she is pregnant. I am a mature seventeen-year-old and she is fifteen. We both want our baby and are willing to assume the responsibilities of parenthood. Neither set of parents will give their consent for us to be married. How can we convince them that we can be responsible and loving parents?

signed,
Rick

Dear Vicki,

All my life I have dreamed of being married and carrying the child of the man I love. Then I met Michael and fell in love. He is extremely possessive and doesn't want to share me with anyone. He even made me get rid of my dog before we got married. How can I convince him that children will enhance our relationship and bring us closer together? I don't feel like a complete woman knowing that I'll never raise a family.

signed,
Cindy

Yours, Mine, and Hers

Numerous legal and ethical issues surround the subject of surrogate childbearing. Is it a form of baby selling, or is it a viable option for individuals who are infertile? What would you decide after reading each situation below?

1. A couple has hired a surrogate and paid all of her expenses. However, the couple and the surrogate both decide they do not want the child. Who should be charged with child abandonment? Should the child be placed in a foster home in the hope of adoption?

2. What should be the legal rights of the surrogate mother if she decides she wants to keep the baby?

3. Prenatal tests indicate that the baby is mentally retarded. The couple wants to abort the pregnancy, but the surrogate says that an abortion is against her religion. Should the couple have the right to terminate the pregnancy without the consent of the surrogate?

4. Prenatal tests reveal a fetal abnormality, and the surrogate wants to terminate the pregnancy. The couple says they are willing to accept the child "as is" and want the pregnancy to continue. Should the surrogate have the right to terminate the pregnancy without the consent of the couple?

5. A single man wants to have children and decides to use a surrogate mother because adoption agencies won't let single men adopt. Should single men have the right to use a surrogate?

6. A prominent female researcher wants to have children and is fertile. However, she does not want to go through the nine-month pregnancy. Should a fertile individual have the right to use a surrogate as a matter of "convenient" childbearing?

Reviewing Important Concepts

1. Trace the development of the neural tube. What is its function?

2. What are some presumptive, probable, and positive signs of pregnancy?

3. Why would a woman choose a midwife for prenatal care and delivery?

4. Differentiate between a certified nurse-midwife and a lay midwife. Why do lay midwives exist?

5. Describe the effects of fetal alcohol syndrome (FAS) on the fetus.

6. What are the dangers of X rays to an ovum?

7. Summarize the effects of rubella on a fetus. How can the congenital rubella syndrome be avoided by a woman who has not had rubella?

8. Briefly describe the developing fetus at four-week intervals.

9. At how many weeks of development does the survival of a premature infant become possible? Why?

10. Describe childbirth, including the stages of labor and what occurs during each stage.

11. Identify five ways to make labor more pleasant.

12. Why is the transition phase the hardest and most uncomfortable phase of labor?

13. Identify problems during delivery associated with drug use by the mother. How do the residual effects of drugs affect the bonding between mother and child?

14. Compare and contrast the Lamaze natural childbirth technique with traditional childbirth. Which technique is more advantageous and why?

15. Why is the Leboyer birthing technique referred to as "birth without violence"?

16. Explain what is meant by an Apgar score of 4. What is the maximum score on this test and when is it given?

17. What is a cesarean section? When should it be performed? Describe the controversy surrounding it.

18. Why are condoms, foams, and jellies the safest and most effective methods of conception control during the postpartum period?

19. When may intercourse resume after delivery? Why?

20. What are the advantages and disadvantages of breast-feeding? How does breast-feeding affect a woman's fertility?

21. Describe when and how amniocentesis is performed. What are some of the major disorders that can be detected using this process?

22. Under what circumstances is amniocentesis or chorionic villus biopsy recommended?

23. Why is a chorionic villus biopsy superior to amniocentesis?

24. When is genetic counseling appropriate, and what may it accomplish?

25. Identify four factors responsible for fertility problems. How can each of these factors be minimized?

26. Identify five causes of female infertility. How can each of these be treated?

27. Identify five causes of male infertility. How can each of these be treated?

28. Compare and contrast home births, hospital births, and birthing center births.

29. What are some of the problems associated with the new developments in reproductive technology?

Self-Discovery

1. The advantages of having children are . . . , but the disadvantages are . . .

2. The advantages of *not* having children are . . . , but the disadvantages are . . .

3. **I want** to become a parent because . . .

   a. I would like the sex of my first child to be a . . . because . . .

   b. Ultimately, I would like to have . . . boys and . . . girls because . . .

   c. To me, quality time with my child means . . .

   d. The advantages of having a child when I am in my mid-thirties as compared to mid-twenties are . . .

   e. The disadvantages of having a child when I am in my mid-thirties as compared to my mid-twenties are . . .

4. **I do *not* want** to become a parent because . . .

5. Explain to your five-year-old where babies come from.

6. What criteria would you use to select your obstetrician/gynecologist?

7. In the future, do you think that a child born with birth defects will sue his or her parents for inadequate prenatal care?

8. How can we lower the infant mortality rate among blacks?

9. Would you want to know the sex of your unborn child before delivery? Why or why not?

10. Where would you choose to have your baby: in a hospital, in a birthing center, or at home? Why?

11. Under what circumstances would you use a nurse-midwife?

12. Should fathers place their priority on career or family? Why?

13. What do you feel is the effect of a baby on a couple's marriage?

14. Should couples curtail their sexual activity with children in the house because they make "noise" during their lovemaking?

15. Should premature infants born before twenty-seven weeks and weighing less than 1000 grams be kept alive through complex and expensive medical technology? Explain.

16. How would you feel if your child was born with the following:

    a. Down's syndrome
    b. Herpes
    c. AIDS
    d. Fetal alcohol syndrome
    e. Spina bifida

17. You are an obstetrician in a small, rural hospital with limited medical equipment and personnel. Because of complications on the operating table, you must decide whose life you will save—the mother's or the unborn child's. What would you decide and why?

18. If you or your partner were infertile, which of the following options would you try and why: (a) artificial insemination, (b) *in vitro* fertilization, (c) fertility drugs, (d) adoption, or (e) surrogate childbearing?

19. Should recipients of donated sperm be allowed to select the donor? Why or why not?

20. Craig regularly donated sperm to the local sperm bank. Should his "children" be considered legal "heirs" to his estate? Defend your answer from Craig's viewpoint and the children's viewpoint.

21. Should the name and medical history of any donor be made available to the child after he or she reaches eighteen years of age?

22. How will research on embryos up to fourteen days old affect the number of pregnancies and abortions in the future?

Self-Quizzes

How well do you know this material? Test yourself by answering the following sample questions.

True/False

____ 1. A female should have a physical examination prior to any attempt to get pregnant.

____ 2. A woman should begin watching her diet and abstain from drugs as soon as her pregnancy is confirmed.

_____ 3. An embryo is as sensitive to drugs in the last trimester as it is in the first.

_____ 4. The number of sperm in an ejaculation is not related to the success rate of conception.

_____ 5. The fertilized ovum is not referred to as a fetus until after the eighth week of development.

_____ 6. Capacitation, or changes that sperm undergo while traveling through the uterus and fallopian tubes, is not necessary for successful fertilization.

_____ 7. The presence of HCG (human chorionic gonadotropin) in a woman's blood or urine is a reliable indicator of pregnancy.

_____ 8. The bloodstreams of the mother and fetus do not mix.

_____ 9. Harmful chemicals and disease agents cannot be transmitted from mother to fetus.

_____ 10. There is no link between the placenta and the mammary glands.

_____ 11. The bag of waters is formed by a fusion of both amniotic and chorionic membranes.

_____ 12. It is not possible for one mature ovum, fertilized by a single sperm, to completely separate into two embryos during development.

_____ 13. Alcohol is considered to be the number one cause of preventable birth defects in the United States.

_____ 14. It is never necessary to use contraception during pregnancy.

_____ 15. Rh factor incompatability may threaten a fetus when an Rh negative woman has several Rh positive babies.

_____ 16. Sexually transmitted diseases and ectopic pregnancies have no relation to each other.

_____ 17. Ninety-five percent of all embryos that implant are successfully carried to term.

_____ 18. The infant mortality rate of whites is almost double that of blacks.

_____ 19. A couple should abstain from sexual intercourse during the last trimester of pregnancy.

_____ 20. An episiotomy is performed more often in hospital deliveries than in birthing center deliveries.

Fill in the Blanks

1. A full-term pregnancy usually lasts about _____ days.

2. Once cell division begins, the zygote is known as a(n) _____ .

3. _____ has occurred when the blastocyst attaches to the endometrium.

4. The organ through which the developing embryo or fetus obtains nourishment and oxygen from its mother's blood is known as the _____ .

5. After about the third month of pregnancy, the placenta becomes a source of large amounts of _____ and _____ .

6. The four positive signs of pregnancy are _____ , _____ , _____ , and _____ .

7. A weight gain of _____ to _____ pounds is associated with the most favorable outcome of pregnancy.

8. Three adverse effects of smoking to the fetus are _____ , _____ , and _____ .

9. The three stages of labor are _____ , _____ , and _____ .

10. Three methods that can be used to treat infertility are _____ , _____ , and _____ .

Answer Key to Self-Quizzes

True/False

1. T	6. F	11. T	16. F
2. F	7. T	12. F	17. F
3. F	8. T	13. T	18. F
4. F	9. F	14. F	19. F
5. T	10. F	15. T	20. T

Fill in the Blanks

1. 266
2. embryo
3. Implantation
4. placenta
5. estrogen and progesterone
6. fetal heartbeat, fetal movement, sonographic recognition of fetus, X-ray confirmation of fetal skeleton
7. twenty, twenty-seven
8. lower birth weight, reduced oxygen-carrying capacity, reduced blood flow through the placenta
9. beginning of labor, birth of the baby, delivery of the placenta
10. *in vitro* fertilization, artificial insemination, ovulation-stimulating hormones

19 Variations in Sexual Behavior

What is unusual sexual behavior? We can answer this question in two different ways. First, if someone defines usual sexual behavior, then we know that any behavior that does not fit that definition is unusual. Or we can turn to the American Psychiatric Association's *Diagnostic and Statistical Manual of Mental Disorders,* Third Edition, Revised (DSM III), and look under psychosexual disorders for what is classified as a variance.

However, human sexual behavior is varied, complex, and constantly changing. What is unacceptable one day may be perfectly acceptable at another time and place. Even the definitions in the DSM have changed with each edition.

What Is Normal?

Assign a behavior rating and indicate the legal sanction for each of the following sexual behaviors by circling the appropriate letters.

Behavior Rating	**Legal Sanction**
N = Normal behavior	MT = Misdemeanor, requires therapy
A = Abnormal behavior	MS = Misdemeanor, requires short-term jail sentence
ED = Emotionally disturbed	F = Felony, requires long-term jail sentence

Behavior	Behavior Rating			Legal Sanction		
1. Frottage	N	A	ED	MT	MS	F
2. Pyromania	N	A	ED	MT	MS	F
3. Masochism	N	A	ED	MT	MS	F
4. Coprophilia	N	A	ED	MT	MS	F
5. Necrophilia	N	A	ED	MT	MS	F
6. Promiscuity	N	A	ED	MT	MS	F
7. Transvestism	N	A	ED	MT	MS	F
8. Copralalia	N	A	ED	MT	MS	F
9. Zoophilia	N	A	ED	MT	MS	F
10. Fetishism	N	A	ED	MT	MS	F
11. Paraphilia	N	A	ED	MT	MS	F
12. Incest	N	A	ED	MT	MS	F
13. Pedophilia	N	A	ED	MT	MS	F
14. Voyeurism	N	A	ED	MT	MS	F
15. Exhibitionism	N	A	ED	MT	MS	F
16. Klismaphilia	N	A	ED	MT	MS	F
17. Sadism	N	A	ED	MT	MS	F
18. Troilism	N	A	ED	MT	MS	F

Can You Decide?

Taking the eighteen sexual behaviors listed on the previous page, place the number of each behavior on the rung of the ladder in order of acceptability.

Most acceptable behavior
for me to engage in

Most acceptable behavior
for someone else to engage in

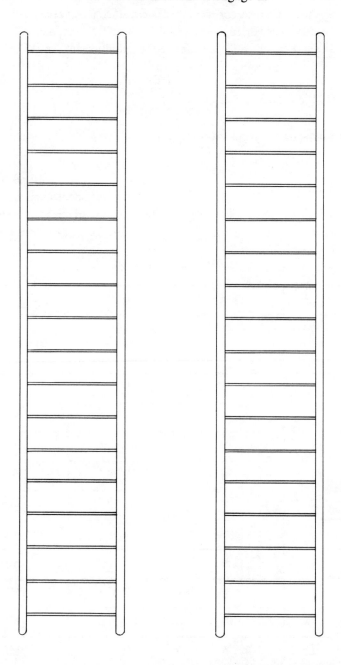

Least acceptable behavior
for me to engage in

Least acceptable behavior
for someone else to engage in

Compare and contrast the ratings on both ladders. Did you rate any of the behaviors differently for yourself and someone else? Why?

Reviewing Important Concepts

1. Distinguish between the various definitions of normal sexual behavior on the basis of the following standards: (a) social, (b) statistical, (c) psychological, (d) legal, (e) moral, (f) phylogenetic, and (g) cultural. Keeping in mind these seven standards, what criteria would you use to characterize abnormal sexual behavior?

2. How do sexual paraphilias differ from sexual dysfunctions?

3. Profile the typical pedophile and identify the type of sexual behavior that occurs. What roles do alcohol and physical violence play in child molestation?

4. How does incest differ from child molestation? Identify and explain three arguments for the incest taboo.

5. Identify the high-risk factors associated with a potential incestuous home.

6. What is the incidence of sexual contact between siblings as compared to father-daughter incest? Why is brother-sister incest less traumatic to the participants than parent-child incest?

7. Distinguish between fetishistic sexual behavior and behavior that is viewed as a paraphilia.

8. With nudity so prevalent in the media and live entertainment, what factors might precipitate an individual to become a voyeur?

9. How does the transvestite differ from the female impersonator and the transsexual?

10. Contrast the profile of the obscene telephone caller with the exhibitionist.

11. Describe hypersexuality. Why may a person who enjoys frequent intercourse feel confident that he or she is not hypersexual?

Self-Discovery

1. Do you feel that incestuous relationships cause deterioration of genetic quality in children through the inheritance of recessive traits? Why or why not?

2. Should marriage and reproduction between adult family members be a legal issue or a matter of personal choice? Explain.

3. Name some objects that you might consider a personal fetish. How do you feel when you are near them?

4. Where would you draw the line between voyeurism and "normal looking"?

5. Why do you feel paraphilias are more common in men than women?

6. Dave and Cindy were placed in an orphanage at fourteen months and two months of age, respectively, after both parents were killed in an automobile accident. Cindy was adopted and raised in Chicago. Dave was adopted and grew up with his new family in Spokane. Both individuals ended up working for the same large corporation and eventually met, fell in love, and wanted to get married. Should they be allowed to get married? Is this incest? Would your answer be different if they did not plan on having any children?

Self-Quizzes

How well do you know this material? Test yourself by answering the following sample questions.

True/False

_____ 1. Sexual behaviors that are considered "normal" or "natural" in our society often differ from those of other cultures and other historical periods.

_____ 2. Many paraphiliacs do not see themselves as ill.

_____ 3. Girls who are victims of sexual abuse are more likely than boys to report episodes of sexual abuse.

_____ 4. The majority of abusive parents come from low-income backgrounds and overcrowded housing.

_____ 5. The typical pedophile is a male in his thirties.

_____ 6. A more severe psychological trauma is likely to result in a child who has been sexually victimized when parents react hysterically rather than calmly.

_____ 7. Incestuous father-daughter relationships continue for a rather long time because the daughter is sexually and romantically attracted to her father.

_____ 8. Aggressive sexual behavior between siblings is indicative of a deep-rooted problem.

_____ 9. According to Gebhard, a preference can be distinguished from a true fetish when a person's sexual preference is something preferred as a substitute over a living sexual partner.

_____ 10. The sale of fetishes has been on a steady decline during the past decade.

_____ 11. Sexual contact with animals is most common among adolescent males from rural areas.

_____ 12. The danger and risk of getting caught appears to be sexually arousing to the voyeur and exhibitionist.

_____ 13. Nymphomaniacs account for more arrests than any other paraphiliacs.

_____ 14. Those who make obscene telephone calls are more of a nuisance than they are criminals.

_____ 15. Most transvestites work in traditionally feminine occupations.

_____ 16. Necrophilia indicates a serious psychological disturbance or a psychotic person.

_____ 17. The use of psychotherapy has been very effective in modifying paraphilics.

_____ 18. Aversion therapy attempts to couple unpleasant experiences with an inappropriate sexual behavior.

_____ 19. Antiandrogens temporarily lower the sex drive in males and thus reduce the compulsiveness of the paraphilia.

_____ 20. Indiscriminate, transient sexual intercourse with many people for the relief of sexual tensions rather than for any feelings of affection is referred to as hypersexuality.

Matching

Match the name of each variant sexual behavior with its definition by placing the correct letter in each blank.

_____ 1. Arousal through sexual activity with a corpse

_____ 2. Wearing the clothes of the opposite sex to obtain sexual arousal

_____ 3. Arousal from prepubertal children

_____ 4. Sexual contact with animals

_____ 5. Arousal from rubbing against someone in a crowded situation

_____ 6. Sexual arousal from the use of nonliving objects

_____ 7. Sexual pleasure from inflicting pain on one's partner

_____ 8. Arousal from watching one's partner have sex with someone else

_____ 9. Sexual pleasure from an enema

_____ 10. Intercourse between persons forbidden by law to marry

_____ 11. Viewing unsuspecting people in the act of disrobing

_____ 12. Arousal from viewing feces

_____ 13. Strong sexual desire that receives no gratification from numerous partners

_____ 14. Sexual pleasure from receiving pain

_____ 15. Sexual pleasure from exposing one's genitals to an unwilling observer

_____ 16. Indiscriminate sexual activity

_____ 17. Using or hearing lewd language

_____ 18. Sexual actions not based on the usual affectionate relationship

_____ 19. An excessive female sex drive

_____ 20. An unchecked impulse to set fires

A. frottage
B. pyromania
C. masochism
D. coprophilia
E. necrophilia
F. hypersexuality
G. promiscuity
H. transvestism
I. coprolalia
J. zoophilia
K. fetishism
L. paraphilia
M. incest
N. pedophilia
O. voyeurism
P. exhibitionism
Q. klismaphilia
R. sadism
S. nymphomania
T. troilism

Answer Key to Self-Quizzes

True/False

1. T	6. T	11. T	16. T
2. T	7. F	12. T	17. F
3. F	8. T	13. F	18. T
4. F	9. T	14. T	19. T
5. T	10. F	15. F	20. F

Matching

1. E	6. K	11. O	16. G
2. H	7. R	12. D	17. I
3. N	8. T	13. F	18. L
4. J	9. Q	14. C	19. S
5. A	10. M	15. P	20. B

20 The Commercialization of Sex

Archaeologists have uncovered pictorial and written representations of human sexuality dating back centuries. As the twentieth century began, a multitude of laws were enacted in an effort to define pornography, obscenity, and erotica. If you were to ask the average American to define these terms, he or she could not do so. However, most individuals would also reply: "I know it when I see it!"

Television Ratings

Using the rating system of the Motion Picture Association of America, rate each of the following television programs and briefly justify your answer. The ratings are G (general audiences, all ages), PG (parental guidance), PG13 (parental guidance for anyone under 13), R (no one under 17 admitted without parent), and X (no one under 17 admitted).

1. "My Two Dads" _____
2. "The Young and the Restless" _____
3. "Cheers" _____
4. "Family Ties" _____
5. "Dallas" _____
6. "Geraldo" _____
7. "Saturday Night Live" _____
8. "Cosby Show" _____
9. "L.A. Law" _____
10. "Donahue" _____
11. "Roseanne" _____
12. "Golden Girls" _____
13. "Knot's Landing" _____
14. "Guiding Light" _____
15. "Late Night with David Letterman" _____
16. "As the World Turns" _____
17. "Our House" _____
18. "thirtysomething" _____
19. "Falcon Crest" _____
20. "General Hospital" _____

You Be the Judge

It has been said that beauty is in the eye of the beholder. Does this also apply to trying to decide whether or not something is pornographic? Label each of the following as erotic, pornographic, or obscene. Compare your answers with those of your friends.

P = Pornographic	O = Obscene	E = Erotic

____ 1. A nude male centerfold in a magazine

____ 2. An X-rated adult movie at the drive-in theater

____ 3. A heterosexual couple engaging in sexual intercourse

____ 4. A homosexual couple engaging in oral sex

____ 5. An eight-year-old girl engaging in intimate sexual behavior with a thirty-year-old man

____ 6. A nude statue in an art exhibit

____ 7. A nude adult male being tied to a chair by his female partner

____ 8. An elderly couple French kissing on a park bench

____ 9. A nude beach

____ 10. Skinny dipping in the river with your partner

____ 11. A male spanking the bare buttocks of his female partner

____ 12. Two females engaging in intimate sexual behavior with a male

____ 13. A heterosexual couple engaging in oral sex

____ 14. Men and women naked in a hot tub together

____ 15. A two-year-old boy and girl exploring each other's bodies in the bathtub

____ 16. A father showering with his inquisitive four-year-old daughter

____ 17. Receiving a massage from a topless masseuse or masseur

____ 18. Watching an adult video at home with your partner

____ 19. A nude female centerfold in a magazine

____ 20. Reading an explicit account of someone else's sexual encounters

Reviewing Important Concepts

1. Describe the typical prostitute. What are some of the early experiences that many prostitutes share?

2. How do the laws exploit prostitutes and sometimes prevent them from leaving the "profession"?

3. Define the Immigration and Nationality Act and the Mann (White Slave) Act.

4. Explain the effect that legalization and decriminalization would have on prostitution.

5. Why is prostitution described as a "victimless" crime? Who is the victim and who is the criminal in the eyes of our current legal system?

6. Explain the 1984 federal Child Protection Act. What was the U.S. Supreme Court's ruling in *New York* v. *Ferber,* 1982? How did this ruling distinguish between obscene materials and child pornography?

7. Compare the television, film, cable, and home video industries in the showing of sexually explicit material.

8. What are the advantages and disadvantages of a woman's posing for nude pictures?

9. What shifts occurred in public attitudes toward pornography between the Commission on Pornography reports of 1970 and 1986?

10. Compare and contrast the conclusions of the 1970 and 1986 Commission on Pornography reports. Why did Congress reject the recommendations of the 1970 report?

11. In *Roth* v. *United States* (1957), the U.S. Supreme Court ruled that in order to be obscene, pornographic material must meet three criteria. List these criteria. Define *prurient interest.*

12. According to *Roth* v. *United States,* did the Comstock Act violate the First Amendment? What did the U.S. Supreme Court rule in regard to freedom of speech and obscenity?

Self-Discovery

1. If prostitution were decriminalized and legalized, how would this change the lives of prostitutes? Would more women become prostitutes? Explain.

2. Do women attend male strip shows for the same reasons that men attend female ones? If so, what are the reasons? If not, why not?

3. Think of your favorite recording artist. Do any of the lyrics he or she sings have a sexual theme? If so, describe the lyrics and their possible effect on sexual behavior.

4. List your five favorite television programs. The next time you watch each one, write down all of the statements, scenes, or commercials that have a sexual connotation. Would you classify each as erotic, pornographic, or obscene?

5. Should men who visit prostitutes be prosecuted as vigorously as prostitutes are? Why or why not? Should a client's name be listed in the newspaper when he is charged?

6. Keeping in mind the arguments for and against the obscenity laws, do you believe that these laws should be retained or abolished? Why?

Self-Quizzes

How well do you know this material? Test yourself by answering the following questions.

True/False

_____ 1. Prostitution is defined as a "profession" of people who perform sexual acts with others free of charge.

_____ 2. The average age for beginning involvement in prostitution is seventeen.

_____ 3. The streetwalker is the most respected of all prostitutes.

_____ 4. Male prostitutes who perform their sexual acts for pay with homosexuals are known as hustlers.

____ 5. Much like the female, the male prostitute is able to perform sexually even though not sexually aroused.

____ 6. There is no correlation between prostitution and troubled homes.

____ 7. Women remain in prostitution out of fear, drug use, low self-esteem, or the need for a pimp's management.

____ 8. Some men visit prostitutes because of a fear of intimacy.

____ 9. Prostitution is legal in most states and is referred to as a "victimless" crime.

____ 10. Erotica and pornography are synonymous.

____ 11. Experimenting with sex as they grow up, males learn that sex is power.

____ 12. Pornographic fantasies have no influence on the defining of values, the molding of personality, or the shaping of behavior.

____ 13. Child pornography is sometimes referred to as "chicken porn."

____ 14. Although child pornography involves children of both sexes, much of it concentrates on boys between eight and ten years of age.

____ 15. The advent of the VCR has had no noticeable effect on the number of people who view sexually explicit films.

____ 16. Pornography that emphasizes aggressive behavior by males toward females has no effect on a man's aggressive attitude.

____ 17. Rapists appear to be aroused by both forced and consenting sex depictions.

____ 18. Public protest against pornography has come primarily from male activist groups.

____ 19. The Supreme Court has legally defined obscenity and now allows communities to set their own standards on obscenity.

____ 20. Erotica is about sexuality, while pornography is about power and sex as a weapon.

Fill in the Blanks

1. The manager of a prostitute's affairs is known as a(n) _____ .

2. The most highly paid of the female prostitutes is called a(n) _____ .

3. A male heterosexual prostitute is often referred to as a(n) _____ .

4. Four patterns of procuring women into prostitution are _____ , _____ , _____ , and _____ .

5. _____ is defined as the depiction of erotic behavior through the written word and pictures with the intent of causing sexual excitement.

6. _____ involves receiving sexual gratification from both giving and receiving pain.

7. People who are involved in child pornography are known as _____ .

8. Three areas in which media eroticization have occurred are _____ , _____ , and _____ .

9. The term _____ refers to commercial ads and messages that are flashed onto a screen so rapidly that a person's mind is not consciously aware of them.

10. _____ is a mutually pleasurable expression between people who have enough power to be there by positive choice.

Answer Key to Self-Quizzes

True/False

1. F	6. F	11. T	16. F
2. T	7. T	12. F	17. T
3. F	8. T	13. T	18. F
4. T	9. F	14. T	19. T
5. F	10. F	15. F	20. T

Fill in the Blanks

1. pimp
2. call girl
3. gigolo
4. befriending, false advertising, purchasing, kidnapping
5. Pornography
6. Sadomasochism
7. pedophiles
8. Magazines, movies, TV
9. *subliminal advertising*
10. Erotica

21 Power and Violence in Sexuality

"Power, like a desolating pestilence, pollutes whate'er it touches." These words of nineteenth-century English poet Percy Bysshe Shelley illustrate vividly the potentially devastating effect power can have on sexual interaction. All too often the desire to dominate, to cast into submission, results in feelings of tenderness and love being replaced by those of force and violence. When these various expressions of emotion get out of balance to the point of being harmful, we must turn to our legal system to determine what is appropriate or inappropriate sexual behavior.

Sexual Practices and the Law

Where would you place the following sexual behaviors and practices on the continuum below? Write the number of the practice or behavior at the appropriate place along the continuum.

---------------- X ----------------------------- X ------------------------------ X ------------------------------- X ----------------

| Prohibited by law | Regulated by law | Freely allowed no legal restrictions | A matter of private decision |

1. Public nudity
2. Sex education in public schools
3. Statutory rape
4. Child pornography
5. Prostitution (male/female)
6. Adultery
7. Interracial sex
8. Incest
9. Homosexual solicitation
10. Voyeurism

11. Exhibitionism
12. Surrogate motherhood
13. Rape
14. Research on frozen embryos
15. Production of pornography
16. Divorce
17. Transsexualism
18. Adult movie theaters
19. Sadomasochism
20. Oral-genital sex

21. Abortion
22. Polygamy
23. Masturbation
24. Eroto-grams
25. Sterilization
26. Cross dressing
27. *In vitro* fertilization
28. Sale of birth control devices
29. Consenting adult sexual behavior
30. Homosexual teachers

Violence in Sex

Complete this questionnaire by indicating the degree to which you agree or disagree with each of the statements, using the scale below. There are no correct or incorrect responses to these statements.

Strongly Agree	Agree	Disagree	Strongly Disagree
1	2	3	4

1. A man walking alone at 11:00 P.M. on a well-lighted, busy street is rarely the victim of sexual violence. 1 2 3 4

2. Women provoke rape by their physical appearance or behavior. 1 2 3 4

3. Pornography depicted in the media causes violent sex crimes. 1 2 3 4

4. Men are rarely the victims of sexual harassment at the workplace. 1 2 3 4

5. Rapists have an uncontrollable sex drive.   1 2 3 4

6. Sadomasochistic behavior is more common in private than research indicates.   1 2 3 4

7. Sex education should be introduced in kindergarten.   1 2 3 4

8. Men who commit rape may come from any race, religion, or social class.   1 2 3 4

9. The majority of rapes occur indoors.   1 2 3 4

10. A man should not be charged with rape if the victim is his wife.   1 2 3 4

11. Statutory rape laws discriminate against men.   1 2 3 4

12. Hitchhiking is safe provided a woman or child is in the car.   1 2 3 4

13. Resisting an attacker will promote homocidal violence.   1 2 3 4

14. Convicted sex offenders should be castrated upon their second conviction.   1 2 3 4

15. Rapes that occur in prisons are due to homosexual tendencies that have been suppressed.   1 2 3 4

16. In the majority of incest cases, the victim reports the attack to an adult who ignores the charges.   1 2 3 4

17. The majority of men who are brought to trial for rape are never convicted on that charge.   1 2 3 4

18. It is more traumatic for the rape victim if she knows her assailant than if she is attacked by a total stranger.   1 2 3 4

19. A man cannot be raped against his will by a female.   1 2 3 4

20. A majority of women who charge rape by a date initially consent to the sexual behavior and later change their mind.   1 2 3 4

21. A nonviolent sexual attack is less traumatic for the victim than is a brutal, violent attack.   1 2 3 4

22. A young black female is more likely to be raped than a young white female.   1 2 3 4

23. College students (male and female) may be the victims of sexual harassment in the classroom.   1 2 3 4

24. A male who is sexually assaulted is less likely to report it than a female who is sexually assaulted.   1 2 3 4

25. A rape victim's previous sexual experience with people other than the defendant should be permissible evidence in a trial.   1 2 3 4

Have You Ever . . .

One of the major problems men and women have is how to interpret signals—a smile, wink, tight jeans, tickling, playing with each other's hair—as sexual or nonsexual behavior. Men and women view male-female relationships differently, and this miscommunication often leads to an unpleasant situation. Read each question below and determine whether or not you have been in a similar situation.

	Yes	No
a. been sexually harassed?	___	___
b. been sexually assaulted/raped?	___	___
c. had your partner misinterpret the level of sexual intimacy you desired?	___	___
d. had sexual intercourse even though you didn't want to because your partner threatened to end your relationship?	___	___
e. had sexual intercourse even though you didn't want to because you felt pressured by your partner's continual arguments?	___	___
f. engaged in kissing or petting because your partner used some degree of physical force when you didn't cooperate?	___	___
g. had sexual intercourse because your partner threatened to use physical force if you didn't cooperate?	___	___
h. had sexual intercourse because your partner used some degree of physical force?	___	___
i. engaged in oral or anal sex when you didn't want to because your partner used threats or physical force?	___	___
j. been sexually assaulted/raped?	___	___

1. Did you answer yes to any of the preceding questions? If so, describe the circumstances.

2. Would better communication in the above circumstance(s) have prevented it (them)? Why or why not?

3. Did you answer no to questions *b* and *j* but yes to questions *d* through *i*? If so, how do you define date rape?

4. If you answered no to question *b* but yes to question *j*, what changed your mind?

Reviewing Important Concepts

1. Briefly summarize the steps that a victim of sexual harassment should take if she or he wants to fight back.

2. Your professor has asked you out to dinner on several occasions and you have said no. Yesterday, when you turned in your midterm exam, he or she asked you again and indicated that you needed to do very well on this exam in order to pass the course. What legal recourse do you have as a student? Identify three organizations that could help you.

3. Explain three different theories that identify the possible causes of sadomasochism.

4. Identify three myths regarding rape and explain why each is false.

5. Why do some men believe that it is acceptable to use physical and psychological force on women who are unwilling to have sex with them?

6. Briefly describe ten ways to reduce the chances of stranger rape.

7. Summarize five ways to reduce the chances of acquaintance rape.

8. Under what circumstances would it be advisable to resist an assailant and fight back? Under what circumstances would it be inadvisable to resist an assailant? Why?

9. Identify five ways in which a rape victim may effectively attack her assailant. Describe the victim who may survive the attack.

10. Describe the emotional aftermath of rape for the victim. Discuss the four emotional phases that she may experience over time.

11. Discuss the reactions of male rape victims as compared to female rape victims.

Self-Discovery

1. Have you ever been the victim of sexual harassment? Describe the situation, your feelings, and how you handled the person who harassed you.

2. Why have women tolerated sexual harassment in the workplace? Is this trend changing? Why or why not?

3. Outline the sexual harassment policy on your campus.

4. Does a woman have the right to decide if and when she will have sex? Does she have the right to change her mind? Does she have the right to choose which sexual behaviors she will engage in? Defend your answers.

5. Should the U.S. Supreme Court decide on an age of consent for all of the states or should the statutory rape laws be abolished? Explain.

6. Why are male rape victims much more likely to be gang raped, beaten, and held longer than female victims? Why would a male victim report being beaten or robbed but not sexually assaulted?

7. Since men are much less likely than women to be the victims of rape, how can we help men deal with the emotional trauma if they have been victimized?

8. Do you feel that there is a direct correlation between violent pornography and sexual assault? Why or why not?

9. You have just come home for a quick lunch and discover your thirteen-year-old daughter crying uncontrollably in the kitchen. After a long silence, she tells you that one of your employees was delivering a package and sexually assaulted her. Keeping in mind your daughter's best interests, answer the following questions:

   a. Would you call the police and report the assault?
   b. Would you call your family physician or take her to the local hospital's emergency room?
   c. Would you contact anyone else?
   d. How would you deal with your employee?
   e. Would you encourage your daughter to press charges and testify in a courtroom?
   f. How would you emotionally support her through this ordeal?
   g. How would you deal with your own emotions?
   h. What would you do if she were pregnant?
   i. Would you move?
   j. Would any of your answers be different if the victim were your spouse? Mother? Sister? If so, why?

10. If a man invites a woman to dinner and the movies, should he expect sex from her in return? If she says no to sex, is he entitled to use force to obtain it? Explain.

11. If your date used physical or psychological force and you engaged in intimate sexual behavior, would you report the assault? Why or why not?

12. How is rape depicted in the media? Is it ever romanticized or eroticized? Give examples of television programs or movies. How is the rapist portrayed? How is the life of the victim subsequently altered and portrayed?

Self-Quizzes

How well do you know this material? Test yourself by answering the following sample questions.

True/False

_____ 1. Sexual harassment must involve some form of personal body content—such as touches, pats, pinches.

_____ 2. Sexual harassment always involves a supervisor.

_____ 3. Sexual harassment is repeated, unwelcome sexual attention.

_____ 4. Most researchers believe that only a small fraction of actual rapes that occur are reported.

_____ 5. In order to pursue a sexual harassment claim under Title VII, a victim must report the harassment to his or her state agency and then to the Equal Employment Opportunity Commission and must do so within 180 days.

_____ 6. Students who are victims of sexual harassment have legal resources through Title IX of the federal Education Amendments and Title VII of the Civil Rights Act.

_____ 7. Sadomasochistic acts are considered a threat to a person's life and can be punished by thirty days in jail or a $100 fine.

_____ 8. The central issues of sadism and masochism are submission, power, and the acting out of fantasy.

_____ 9. Rape is a violent crime, not a crime of passion or sex.

_____ 10. The incidence of women falsely accusing a man of rape is the same as for any other felony.

_____ 11. Most rapists are strangers and force fellatio.

_____ 12. Rape victims should seek medical help immediately so that evidence can be preserved.

_____ 13. Sexual violence by adolescents is becoming increasingly common in all communities.

_____ 14. The anger rapist feels sexually inadequate and uses a weapon to intimidate his victim.

_____ 15. The mutilation of the victim by the sadistic rapist occurs in approximately 10 percent of all rapes.

_____ 16. Approximately 45 percent of all rapes occur in the victim's own home or near her home.

_____ 17. In general, males cannot be raped without their consent.

_____ 18. Acquaintance rape usually occurs between the hours of 10:00 P.M. and 2:00 A.M.

_____ 19. Research findings indicate that many young men and women believe that forced sexual intercourse is permissible under certain circumstances.

_____ 20. The logic behind the marital rape shield available in most states is that a wife has "consented" to all sexual acts by her husband.

Fill in the Blanks

1. The real issue in sexual harassment is _____ .

2. _____ is receiving sexual arousal and pleasure by inflicting or receiving physical or emotional pain.

3. Voluntary sexual intercourse between an adult male and a minor female (who is under the age of consent) who are not married to each other is called _____ .

4. The _____ rapist expresses rage by verbal abuse and physical attack.

5. Rape _____ often make prosecution of rapes difficult and cause victims to underreport it.

Answer Key to Self-Quizzes

True/False

1. F	6. T	11. F	16. T
2. F	7. F	12. T	17. F
3. T	8. F	13. T	18. T
4. T	9. T	14. F	19. T
5. T	10. T	15. F	20. T

Fill in the Blanks

1. power
2. Sadomasochism
3. statutory rape
4. anger
5. myths